D0506467

LOOK GREAT
NAKED
DIET

LOOK GREAT
NAKED
DIET

CHANGE YOUR SET POINT,
CHANGE YOUR LIFE

Brad Schoenfeld, CSCS

AVERY
a member of Penguin Group (USA) Inc.
New York

Neither the publisher nor the author is engaged in rendering professional advice or services to the individual reader. The ideas, procedures, and suggestions contained in this book are not intended as a substitute for consulting with your physician. All matters regarding health require medical supervision. Neither the author nor the publisher shall be liable or responsible for any loss, injury, or damage allegedly arising from any information or suggestion in this book. The opinions expressed in this book represent the personal views of the author and not of the publisher.

The recipes contained in this book are to be followed exactly as written. Neither the publisher nor the author is responsible for your specific health or allergy needs that may require medical supervision or for any adverse reactions to the recipes contained in this book.

While the author has made every effort to provide accurate telephone numbers and Internet addresses at the time of publication, neither the publisher nor the author assumes any responsibility for errors or for changes that occur after publication.

Most Avery books are available at special quantity discounts for bulk purchase for sales promotions, premiums, fund-raising, and educational needs. Special books or book excerpts also can be created to fit specific needs. For details, write Penguin Group (USA) Inc. Special Markets, 375 Hudson Street, New York, NY 10014.

a member of
Penguin Group (USA) Inc.
375 Hudson Street
New York, NY 10014
www.penguin.com

Copyright © 2004 by Brad Schoenfeld

All rights reserved. This book, or parts thereof, may not be reproduced
in any form without permission.
Published simultaneously in Canada

Library of Congress Cataloging-in-Publication Data

Schoenfeld, Brad.
Look great naked diet : change your set point, change your life / Brad Schoenfeld.
p.   cm.
Includes bibliographical references and index.
ISBN 1-58333-185-9
1. Reducing diets.   2. Nutrition.   3. Exercise.   4. Health.   I. Title.
RM222.2.S334   2004   2003060085
613.2'5—dc22

Printed in the United States of America
1   3   5   7   9   10   8   6   4   2

This book is printed on acid-free paper. ∞

Book design by Amanda Dewey

Acknowledgments

To super-agent Bob Silverstein, for being not only a terrific agent but also a true friend and mentor.

To John Duff, for seeing the potential in this project and giving it life.

To Eileen Bertelli, for believing in the book and putting in the necessary resources to make it a success.

To Kristen Jennings, for your expert editorial suggestions, helping to trim the book's fat and improve upon its strengths.

To my parents, for instilling in me the importance of critical thinking and taking a scientific approach to life.

To all my clients at the Personal Training Center for Women, past and present, for helping me perfect my program and further my quest for self-actualization.

To all the professors of nutrition and exercise science who, through your teachings and writings, have furthered my knowledge in a complex field.

Contents

Introduction

Congratulations! You have in your hands a book that will change everything you thought you knew about losing body fat and keeping it off permanently. Skeptical? I don't blame you. After all, it seems a new fad diet hits the bookstores on a weekly basis. There are high-carb/low-fat diets, and low-carb/high-fat diets, all-fruit diets, no-fruit diets, even cabbage soup diets! From Atkins to the Zone, diets span the alphabet from A to Z.

The stark reality, though, is that fad diets don't work. While most will induce temporary weight loss, they simply don't provide the ability to sustain this weight loss for an extended period of time. They are short-term solutions to a long-term problem and neglect to address the main issues associated with ongoing weight management. This is reflected in the grim statistics: Fewer than 10 percent of those who go on a diet are able to keep the weight off after a year's time.

Well, rest assured, the Look Great Naked Diet (hereafter referred to as the LGN Diet) isn't just another fad diet. Rather, it's a cutting-edge, scientifically based program that will help you get your body fat down to levels you never dreamed possible and, more important, maintain these results over the long haul. Rather than prescribing a one-size-fits-all cookie-cutter nutritional approach, it shows you how to customize a dietary regimen to your own unique needs and body type. Whether it's losing weight, gaining lean muscle, or simply maintaining optimal health and wellness, you'll be able to manipulate dietary variables to achieve your objective. There are no gimmicks here; just tried and true dietary principles proven to stand the test of time.

I subscribe to the Chinese adage that says: "Give a person a fish and you feed him for a day; teach a person to fish and you feed him for life." Accordingly, my aim is to teach you the physiology behind the diet so that you understand not only what to do, but also why you should do it. Here's a chapter-by-chapter overview of what will be covered:

- *Chapter 1* introduces the concept of body-weight set point and explains its impact on fat storage. You'll see how evolution has made the human body resistant to fat loss and why gender and aging factors compound the problem.
- *Chapter 2* discusses the specific genetic and environmental influences that govern weight management. You'll learn about leptin, the "master hormone" in regulating fat balance, as well as other hormones and enzymes that share secondary roles in the process. And you'll get the lowdown on why people with similar genetics can have dramatically different physiques based on their lifestyle choices.
- *Chapter 3* explains the LGN Diet approach to conquering your set point and enjoying lasting weight management. You'll see how, through proper dietary manipulation, dietary obstacles can be overcome; hunger and appetite can be regulated; metabolic rate can be increased; and environment can be controlled—all by adhering to the program set forth in this book.
- *Chapter 4* details the truth about carbs, explaining their importance in a balanced nutritional regimen and why low-carb diets are unnecessary and often counterproductive to achieving optimal body composition. You'll learn how to choose carbs based on their nutrient density, find out how to manipulate intake based on your body type (a classification system based on body structure), and get a complete rundown of the "best" carb sources.
- *Chapter 5* delves into the complexities of protein. You'll discover why protein is the "king of all nutrients" and needs to be consumed in adequate amounts—significantly more than RDA guidelines—in order to optimize body composition. A specific formula is given for estimating ideal intake and a listing of which protein sources you should eat and which you should avoid is furnished for easy reference.
- *Chapter 6* explores the role of dietary fat in weight management. You'll

learn why low-fat diets don't work over the long haul. There are "good" fats and "bad" fats, and, by choosing the right ones, you can actually accelerate your body's ability to burn fat. A detailed analysis of each type of fat is provided, along with a listing of the best "healthy-fat foods" to consume.

- *Chapter 7* discusses the forgotten nutrient: water. Water doesn't just quench your thirst; it plays an integral part in cellular processes—including the metabolism of body fat and the preservation of basic health. You'll learn how to estimate fluid intake and why certain variables affect how much you need. Suffice it to say, it's not the standard advice to simply drink eight 8-ounce glasses of water a day.

- *Chapter 8* shows how to put together a customized nutritional regimen. Using the principles learned in previous chapters, you'll get complete plans for different physique goals, be it fat loss, weight maintenance, or bulking up (yes, there are some people who actually want to *gain* weight!). Strategies are given on how to avoid diet-related plateaus, and seven-day sample menu plans are provided to illustrate the possibilities for dietary variety.

- *Chapter 9* details expert tips for achieving and maintaining super-low levels of body fat. These tips are at the cutting edge of nutritional science. By incorporating them into your dietary regimen, you'll turn your body into a fat-burning machine, allowing it to operate at peak efficiency.

- *Chapter 10* explores the link between nutrition and exercise. Diet has a profound effect on exercise, from both performance and body composition standpoints. Specific guidelines are given for what to eat before, during, and after a workout so that you achieve optimal results from your training efforts.

- *Chapter 11* outlines a game plan to help you when you're eating away from home. Dining out is the downfall of many a dieter and, if not properly managed, can completely derail your weight-loss efforts. By adhering to the protocol set forth herein, this won't be an issue.

- *Chapter 12* explains how to get your body into top shape for a specific occasion, be it a physique competition, pool party, wedding, or any other single-day event. Using a modified carb-deplete/carb-load regimen, it's a one-week program that's guaranteed to have you looking your very best.

- *Chapter 13* highlights the risks and rewards of taking dietary supplements. Vitamins, minerals, and muscle-building aids are evaluated and, where applicable, specific recommendations for what to take and how much to use are given. It's an unbiased view on a controversial topic that is sure to inform and enlighten.

- *Chapter 14* debunks some of the most common myths associated with nutrition and fat loss. Is there any truth to the recommendation that cardio should be performed first thing in the morning on an empty stomach? No! Is liposuction really a permanent solution for getting rid of your love handles? No! You'll find out why these and many other theories that have somehow been taken as gospel really don't hold up in practice.

- *Chapter 15* contains a collection of delicious, healthy recipes contributed by some of the top fitness models and bodybuilders in the world. These are the favorite recipes of people who make their living by keeping their bodies in top shape. You'll see that eating healthy doesn't have to be boring. Whether it's breakfast, lunch, dinner, or snacks, you'll find recipes that make your mouth water.

In sum, this book is the result of my lifetime interest in fitness and diet. I've been a student of the scientific literature for many years and have applied the concepts presented in the LGN Diet both personally and professionally with tremendous success. If you follow the program as directed, you will achieve your best shape ever—I guarantee it!

THE
PROBLEM
OF DIETING

PART ONE

CHAPTER 1

Body-Fat Blues

We're going to open with a short course on food chemistry. Bear with me on this. It's a little involved, but it's absolutely necessary for understanding the principles that will guide you in your quest to customize an individual diet plan.

To begin with, let's agree that the primary objective of virtually every diet is to reduce body fat—nothing is more detrimental to your physique from an aesthetic standpoint. Fat hangs off your body like loose jelly, obscuring your muscle tone and wreaking havoc on your appearance. Like it or not, slim is in, and most people are willing to go to great lengths to lose their flab.

The health-related consequences of carrying excess weight are staggering, as obesity is responsible for more than 300,000 deaths a year.[1] Obesity is directly correlated with an increased incidence of diabetes, hypertension, and heart disease, and has been implicated in various forms of cancer and other maladies. It accounts for more chronic health problems and a worse quality of life than both poverty and tobacco use![2] Obesity has become an epidemic recognized as one of the top ten global health problems by the World Health Organization.

But keeping body fat to a minimum is easier said than done. Americans spend billions of dollars each year in their quest to win the battle of the bulge.[3] Between nutritionists, dieticians, supplements, and the like, the weight-loss industry produces more goods and services than the gross national product of many third-world nations! Despite these enormous expenditures, however, Americans as a people are losing the war; more than two-thirds of the population remains overweight and out of shape.[4]

FAT FACTS

To most people, body fat is a subject that raises numerous questions. What causes fat to be stored? How is fat burned? Why are some areas of the body more resistant to fat loss than others? To unlock these mysteries, let's take an in-depth look at the physiology of body fat.

It's important to start out by noting that body fat has diverse biological roles: It provides a reserve source of energy, acts as storage site for fat-soluble vitamins, serves as protective padding for your internal organs, and insulates your body against the cold. Researchers estimate that men need to maintain a minimum of about 3 percent body fat to sustain normal bodily function. Since body fat is involved in regulating menstruation, this percentage is significantly higher in women, generally in the 12 percent range.

In mammals, fat is contained in cells called *adipocytes*. Adipocytes are pliable storehouses that either shrink or expand to accommodate fatty deposits and are

Healthy Body-Fat Levels for Women

From a medical perspective, a "healthy" body-fat percentage for men is considered to be 12 to 21 percent while a "healthy" body fat percentage for women is considered to be 18 to 27 percent. Understand, however, that these are generalizations that must be taken in context. There is nothing wrong with having lower body-fat levels as long as it does not interfere with normal body function (in women, body-fat levels below about 12 percent can cause a cessation of menstruation). My advice here is to let the mirror be your guide as to whether you are overfat. The most important thing is to like your body!

present in virtually every part of the body. About 85 percent of an adipocyte is made up of a single fat globule. There is a direct correlation between the size of adipocytes and obesity: the larger your adipocytes, the fatter you appear. However, although adipocytes can be reduced in size, they can't be completely eliminated. The harsh reality is, once adipocytes form, you are basically stuck with them for life.

On the surface of each adipocyte are tiny *receptors* that control the storage and release of fat from the cell. Receptors can be likened to doorways; they either allow fat into or out of adipocytes. There are two basic types of fat receptors: alpha-2 receptors and beta receptors. Taking the doorway analogy a step further, alpha-2 receptors are the "entrances" that let fat into adipocytes for long-term storage while beta receptors are the "exits" that let fat out of adipocytes to be burned for energy. Depending on various physiologic factors (hormonal stimulus, enzymatic activity, caloric availability, etc.), these receptors ultimately determine whether body fat is gained or lost.[5,6]

The accretion of body fat begins while you're in your mother's womb. During the last fetal trimester, there is a dramatic increase in both the size and number of fat cells.[7] This accelerated buildup of body fat continues after birth, with a threefold increase in adipocyte formation until about the age of six. Body-fat levels then level off until puberty, when fat deposition picks up again (especially for women).

After adolescence, body-fat levels tend to rise consistently with age. On average, people gain about 10 percent body fat per decade. This is largely due to an age-related loss of muscle tissue.[8] Beginning as early as the mid-twenties, a person loses roughly one percent of their muscle mass each year and continues to do so throughout the rest of his/her life. Muscle is the most metabolically active tissue in the body; the more muscle you have, the more calories you burn. Thus, a reduction of muscle progressively slows metabolism, causing a gradual but steady increase in body fat.

THE INFLUENCE OF GENDER

Why is it that men seem to lose weight rather easily while women struggle to drop even a few pounds? The answer is related to body-fat distribution. Women tend to be pear-shaped (called a gynecoid physique), with a predisposition to storing fat in the lower body, while men are generally apple-shaped (called an android physique), storing the majority of their fat in the upper body.[9]

What does this have to do with weight gain? Well, it turns out that where you store fat has a direct bearing on how it's metabolized.[10,11] Here's why: In women, the lower body has a much greater ratio of alpha-2 receptors to beta receptors (as high as 6:1, by some estimates).[12] This is in direct opposition to men, where the ratio is about 1:1. (Both sexes have roughly equal distributions in the upper body.) So with all these fat-hungry alpha-2 receptors in the lower body allowing fat into their adipocytes, women are more likely to hoard body fat in this region.

Due to the effects of estrogen, women have an increased propensity to store body fat. Among its many functions, estrogen is integrally involved in the storage of body fat. Specifically, it exerts a regional influence over lipoprotein lipase—an enzyme that assists the body in storing fat.[13] In lower body adipocytes, estrogen stimulates lipoprotein lipase activity, causing fat to readily accumulate in this area.[14] Conversely, estrogen has the opposite effect in the upper body, where it actually suppresses the activity of lipoprotein lipase and thereby impedes fat deposition.[15] This site-specific response, which begins during puberty, diverts fat away from the upper body and into the hips and thighs, producing the rounded features normally associated with the female physique.[16]

When a woman becomes pregnant, body-fat levels rise even further. Fat is a primary energy source used for fetal development and maternal lactation. It helps to nourish the fetus and fuel the growth and maturation of fetal organs, vessels, and bones. In order to support these extra energy requirements, the body attempts to mobilize as much fat as possible. It does so by secreting a large amount of progesterone—a hormone that increases appetite.[17] Progesterone levels remain elevated throughout pregnancy, inducing the intense cravings commonly associated with childbirth. In addition, there is a rapid proliferation of adipocytes. Millions of new fat cells are created, with most of them going directly to the lower body. These effects are compounded with multiple pregnancies; after the second or third child, losing postpartum weight becomes even more problematic.

While it might seem that men are on Easy Street with respect to fat deposition, this isn't the case. Despite having lower levels of body fat and an easier time dropping weight, they are subject to a different problem: Their fat-storage patterns predispose them to a variety of health-related complications. Specifically, abdominal fat is linked to Syndrome X—a multifaceted metabolic disorder that encompasses diabetes (insulin resistance), high cholesterol, and hypertension.[18] This translates into an increased incidence of premature death from cardiovascular disease.

Women are more or less protected from cardiovascular disease until menopause. During this period, changes take place in the body that cause a shift in the distribution of body fat. Without the "benefit" of estrogen to influence fat storage, fat begins to accumulate to a much greater degree in the midsection and the hourglass figure gradually morphs into the male-oriented android shape. And once this happens, women are just as susceptible to heart attacks as men.[19]

THE EVOLUTION OF YOUR SET POINT

The capacity to store fat varies from person to person. Some are able to eat whatever they want without gaining weight while others seem to pack on the pounds just looking at food. What causes these discrepancies? The answer lies in a phenomenon known as set point.

Simply stated, the set point is the body's way of physiologically regulating your weight. Through various processes, there is a coordinated effort by your body to adjust its intake and expenditure of energy so that a specified amount of fat stores are maintained. Any attempt to deviate from this predetermined level is actively resisted.

The regulation of body weight is similar to that of your internal temperature. A change in your temperature is met by appropriate alterations in heat production (i.e., shivering) or heat losses (i.e., sweating) to defend the body's set temperature and return it to a normal level. The major difference here is that while body temperature is more or less the same for all people (approximately 98.6 degrees Fahrenheit), body weight varies significantly between individuals.

The set point theory of body-weight regulation has been scientifically validated. Research carried out on adopted babies shows a high correlation between the body type of adoptees with their biological parents and a low correlation with their adopted parents.[20,21] Similar results are seen in identical twins, who display roughly equal levels of body fat with one another, even when they are raised apart under differing environmental conditions.[22,23] Given the overwhelming evidence, there is little doubt that genetics play a big role in long-term weight management.

Your set point can be traced back to the dawn of humankind. During Paleolithic times (i.e., the caveman era), food was scarce. There were no supermarkets, grocery stores, or restaurants that stocked an assortment of your favorite goodies. If you wanted to eat, you had to fend for yourself. Humans were hunters and gatherers, chasing down wild game with primitive implements and scavenging the wild for nuts and berries. These types of conditions persisted throughout the ages. In the recorded history of the more developed Middle East, Europe, or China, there was never a long period of uninterrupted food abundance, whereas famines were regular and frequent.[24] Days or even weeks could go by without having a meal.

In order to deal with these continual feast-famine cycles, the human body developed a tendency to store food (in the form of body fat) when it was available and then use the fat reserves for fuel during periods of deprivation. This generally followed a seasonal pattern. Our ancestors would fatten up during the warm summer months when there was an abundance of food so that they would have enough stored energy to endure the frigid winter months when food was scarce.

As you might expect, thin people were at a significant disadvantage during periods of extended famine. Without an adequate reserve of fat, they eventually ran out of the energy necessary to sustain bodily functions, ultimately dying off. Those who survived tended to carry "fat genes"—genes that evolved to efficiently store body fat and resist losing it. And it's these same genes that were passed down through the ages and inherited into a large segment of today's population.

Fast-forward to the present: While our genetics haven't changed much, our environment has. In the Western world, famine has been all but wiped out. Anytime you care to eat, be it day or night, an abundance of refined, high-fat, calorie-dense foods are readily available. And everything from burgers to fries to soft drinks are now supersized, so, in addition to the poor quality, there's an excess of quantity—a surefire combination for gaining weight.

Compounding the problem, advances in technology and transportation have drastically reduced the need for physical activity in everyday life. Our jobs are largely sedentary. Instead of doing physical work and hunting for food, we now spend most of our time behind a desk. Television, DVDs, the Internet, and most any of the other indoor activities have eliminated the need to leave our homes for entertainment. The facts are clear: Our bodies still think we are living the lives of our Paleolithic ancestors when, in fact, we have become a nation of inactive couch potatoes.

In the next chapter, you will learn how the body's set point is regulated and how you can use it to effectively manage your weight long term.

CHAPTER 2

Set Point and You

The theory of a body-weight set point goes back to the 1940s when studies on rats revealed that small lesions on a part of the brain called the *hypothalamus* produced dramatic changes in food intake and body weight.[1] Intrigued by this finding, scientists began conducting additional experiments using electrical stimulation. These studies showed that when the lateral aspect of the hypothalamus was electrically stimulated, it triggered excessive eating and drinking. Conversely, electrical stimulation of the ventromedial area of the hypothalamus inhibited consumption of food. This led to the theory that the lateral hypothalamus was the body's "feeding center" and the ventromedial hypothalamus was the body's "satiety center." These centers, it was believed, were the driving forces that regulated set point.

Soon thereafter, however, the theory of "feeding" and "satiety" centers came under scrutiny. Continuing research showed that mice with lesions that would inhibit the function of the ventromedial hypothalamus (the area that signals satiety) were finicky eaters. These mice actually *reduced* food intake when a food was bitter or stale—not exactly the type of behavior you'd expect if their satiety centers were knocked out. Based on this and other information, a new theory emerged: Set point was actually a product of body-fat levels, which somehow signaled the hypothalamus to control appetite.[2] But despite extensive efforts to explain how this process worked, the answer remained elusive for many years.

A major breakthrough came in 1994 when a group of scientists from The Rockefeller University in New York City made a discovery that revolutionized our understanding of body-weight set point. While studying the differences between fat and thin mice, they noticed that certain mice were morbidly obese and couldn't lose weight regardless of how strictly they dieted. Further investigation revealed that these mice had a defective gene (known as the *ob gene*) that interacted with the hypothalamus via a specific hormone.[3] The hormone was called leptin (the name from *leptos*, Greek for "thin"), and, as more and more research came to light, it became apparent that leptin was the missing piece to the body-weight set-point puzzle.

From a weight-management perspective, the discovery of leptin truly was a groundbreaking event. Produced mainly in adipose tissue (fat cells), it acts like a long-term energy gauge for your body. Think of it as a body-weight thermostat—a "lipostat" if you will—that monitors how much fat you have and then continually relays this information to your hypothalamus.[4] The amount of leptin secreted is highly correlated to the amount of body fat you carry, both in the size and number of adipocytes. As a general rule, the fatter you are, the more leptin you secrete.[5,6,7]

Here is an overview of how leptin functions: After being secreted by fat cells, leptin travels through your bloodstream and enters your brain. There, the hypothalamus reads its signal and communicates with other brain centers. These brain centers then compare the amount of fat that you have with the amount of fat you were programmed to have (i.e., your set point) and make adjustments in both appetite and metabolic rate.[8] A decrease in leptin (associated with a loss of body fat)

The Hypothalamus: What You Need to Know

The hypothalamus (*hype*-oh-thal-uh-mus) is a pea-sized region of the brain that controls an immense number of bodily functions as well as influences such behaviors as arousal, rage, aggression, embarrassment, escape from danger, pleasure, copulation, and, most central to the subject of this book, eating and drinking. It is located in the middle of the base of the brain and has two main regions: a lateral (side) aspect and medial (middle) aspect. These regions have different actions (and often opposing actions) and combine to bring homeostasis (a state of balance) to the human body.

jacks up appetite and suppresses metabolism while an increase in leptin (associated with gains in body fat) curbs appetite and elevates metabolism. In this way, body weight is maintained within a fairly narrow range of your set point.

But rather than acting directly on appetite and metabolic rate, leptin exerts its effects by activating other hormones and neurochemicals. These compounds can be grouped into two basic classes: *Orexins*, which stimulate appetite and/or suppress metabolism; and *anorexins*, which promote satiety and/or boost metabolism.[9] (See the appendix for a list of orexins and anorexins.)

LEPTIN IN PRACTICE

When your body's energy levels are in a state of balance (caloric intake is equal to caloric expenditure), leptin is normally secreted in direct proportion to your existing body-fat percentage.[10] But when the body's set point is threatened (such as during severe dieting or fasting), there is an override of normal leptin production, with fluctuations well beyond those predicted solely on changes in fat mass.[11,12] During attempts at weight loss, for instance, a 10 percent reduction in body weight has been shown to cause more than a 50 percent decrease in serum leptin levels.[13] Conversely, a 10 percent weight gain increases leptin in excess of 20 percent.[14] (As you can see, leptin is much more sensitive to weight loss than to weight gain. This makes evolutionary sense since carrying extra body fat was more advantageous to our Paleolithic ancestors than carrying too little.)

Let's take a look at how the actions of leptin translate into practice. Say your set point is 20 percent body fat and, employing a typical calorie-restricted meal plan, you diet down to 12 percent. So far, so good, right? Well, not really, at least over the long term. Perceiving starvation, your body will try to defend against what it believes is a threat to its survival. Leptin levels will fall precipitously, setting off a chain of hormonal and neurochemical events (stimulation of orexins and suppression of

---

The Effects of Leptin

Increase in fat levels → Increase in leptin → Appetite suppression, increase in metabolism

Decrease in fat levels → Decrease in leptin → Increase in appetite, decrease in metabolism

anorexins) that result in an increase in appetite and a reduction in energy expenditure. Consequently, if you want to maintain this new weight, a great deal of resolve will be required to fight off your body's attempt to return to its set point.

RESISTANCE TO LEPTIN

Given the effects of leptin on set point, you'd think its actions would prevent people from gaining excessive amounts of weight (just as it protects against extreme weight loss). This, however, isn't the case. You see, before it can reach the hypothalamus, leptin must first cross the blood-brain barrier (BBB). As the name implies, the BBB is a protective wall that surrounds the brain, selectively allowing certain compounds to pass through while blocking others. For leptin, this process is facilitated by specific transporters, which serve to shuttle leptin across the BBB.

But there's a catch: Leptin has a saturation level above which its uptake into the brain doesn't increase.[15] Exceedingly high levels of leptin place an overload on leptin transporters. Eventually, the transporters become desensitized and lose their ability to carry leptin across the BBB.[16] This phenomenon, called leptin resistance, renders much of the leptin in the bloodstream inconsequential.

Obesity is a primary cause of leptin resistance. When an obese person gains weight, his body increases leptin production in an attempt to prevent further obesity. But after being constantly bombarded by leptin, his leptin transporters lose their sensitivity and the appropriate satiety signals never reach the brain. Thus, while there is a large amount of leptin circulating in the blood, the person's brain thinks that he's much thinner than he actually is and continues to store more fat. This creates a vicious cycle where additional weight gain further desensitizes leptin transporters, inducing further weight gain, and so on.[17]

You don't have to be obese, however, to suffer from leptin resistance. Massive overeating, the effects of aging, and adherence to a high-fat diet are all associated with decreased leptin transport and diminished leptin function.[18,19,20] In all of these cases, increased fat storage, above and beyond set point, is the result.

BEYOND LEPTIN

While leptin appears to be the primary regulator of body-weight set point, it is by no means the only one. Realize that the human body is the most intricate piece of machinery in the world. No device, be it man-made or otherwise, can come close to approximating its intricacies. Accordingly, the pathways controlling food intake have built-in redundancies so that the loss of one signaling system is compensated for by the activation of another.[21] In this way, no single system determines your ultimate fate.

Blood sugar (i.e., blood glucose) is perhaps the most important short-term regulator of set point.[22,23] Blood sugar is derived from the food that you eat. After a meal, your body breaks down carbohydrates (and, to a lesser extent, protein and fats) into glucose (a simple sugar). Under normal circumstances, the glucose molecules then circulate throughout your bloodstream until they're taken up in the cells and used for energy.

Since glucose is a primary source of fuel for many bodily tissues, its levels are under tight bodily control. This task is carried out by, as you may have guessed, the hypothalamus, which contains various nerve cells that monitor the amount of circulating blood glucose. When blood glucose falls below a certain threshold, it sends up a red flag that body fuel stores are threatened.[24] The hypothalamus, in turn, initiates a response similar to the response to falling leptin that increases hunger and slows metabolism. After eating a meal, appropriate glucose levels are quickly reestablished and hunger does not manifest again until glucose levels fall below the given threshold.

The blood glucose system works in conjunction with the pancreatic hormone insulin. Insulin is the primary regulator of blood sugar. When blood sugar levels rise following a meal, the pancreas secretes insulin to drive glucose into target cells. Although its main targets are muscle and fat cells, insulin also acts on the brain, where

Set-Point Regulators

Leptin: Produced mainly in fat cells, leptin is the "master" hormone that regulates body fat. It influences a cascade of hormones that regulate body-weight set point.

Insulin: Secreted by the alpha-cells of the pancreas, insulin is a storage hormone. While its primary function is to clear blood sugar from circulation, it also plays a role in other bodily processes, including the rebuilding of tissue proteins (such as muscle).

Ghrelin: Often referred to as the "hunger molecule," ghrelin is produced in the stomach and has effects that are diametrically opposed to leptin. It is activated when the stomach is empty and causes a slowdown in metabolism and an increase in hunger.

it binds to insulin receptors in the hypothalamus, exerting similar effects to those of leptin (i.e., increased satiety and elevated metabolic rate).[25] Unfortunately, excess insulin can cause unwanted body-fat storage, as will be discussed in great detail in later chapters, so properly managing this hormone is essential to weight control.

Another system involved in set-point regulation is a hormone called ghrelin.[26] Produced in the stomach, ghrelin has been called the "hunger molecule," with effects diametrically opposite those of leptin. When the stomach is empty, ghrelin signals the hypothalamus to slow down fat utilization and jack up hunger. In this way, it acts as a meal-to-meal control system, influencing the onset and termination of food intake.

Food itself has a direct effect on promoting satiety. As nutrients enter the gut, they stimulate various gastrointestinal hormones. While the central role of these hormones is to aid in digestion, they also participate in the control of hunger. Thus, to a certain degree, food serves as its own regulator of meal size.

Food consumption also brings about a phenomenon called the thermic effect of food (TEF). Each time you eat, your body burns off a percentage of the calories consumed during digestion. In a typical mixed meal, this equates to about 10 percent of caloric intake. Hence, for every 500 calories consumed, only about 450 will be assimilated by your body (each macronutrient has a different TEF so the actual amount burned off can be higher or lower depending on the types of foods eaten). Interestingly, TEF can be influenced by body type: those who are obese have a reduced TEF while those who are fit show an increased thermic response to eating.[27,28]

So as you can see, the control of set point is an extremely complex entity. Multiple short-term systems interact in a coordinated effort to augment the long-term effects of leptin, maintaining body-fat levels within predetermined boundaries.

CONQUERING YOUR SET POINT

Based on a rigid interpretation of the set-point theory, it would appear that your body weight is a product of destiny and you are helpless to do anything about it. Thankfully, this isn't the case. To understand why, let's delve a little more into the origins of set point.

It is postulated that your set point is imprinted while you're in your mother's womb.[29] From the moment you are conceived, nature is at work deciding how much fat your body will strive to maintain. This process is unique to each individual. One person might have a set point of, say, 10 percent body fat while another might have one of 30 percent. The exact number is, for the most part, dependent on the genes of your parents.

But your set point isn't static. It continues to evolve after birth and into childhood, shifting in conjunction with various physiologic changes that occur over your life span. For example, it has been well documented that prolonged maintenance of a body weight over your set point can lead to an elevation of your set point.[30,31] This is largely due to the increased number of fat cells associated with weight gain. Once new adipocytes form, your body raises set point to keep them fully stuffed with fat.

Despite this propensity to stockpile fat, however, it is possible to reset your set point at a lower level and this is the focus of the Look Great Naked Diet. With the proper nutritional approach, you can alter various internal mechanisms to convince your body it doesn't need that much fat for sustenance. Provided there is no perceived threat to survival, your body will become amenable to maintaining a reduced weight and you can get leaner than you previously thought possible.

THE IMPACT OF ENVIRONMENT

Up to this point, we've spent a good deal of time discussing the genetic component of body composition. But while genetics certainly play a major role in long-term weight management, a strong environmental component exists, too. In fact, scientists estimate that up to 50 percent of your physique is determined by non-genetic factors—factors that include the influence of family, school, peers, community, time of day, week, and even lunar phase.[32,33,34]

The process begins in childhood where parental behavior shapes food acceptance. To a large degree, this is a function of food availability. It has been shown that early exposure to fruit and vegetables or to foods high in calories, sugar, and fat conditions your preference for, and consumption of, these foods later in life.[35] By having access to only certain taste sensations, you develop a comfort level with certain foods and not others.

Throughout the early years, psychological factors also play a role in shaping your attitude toward diet. For example, if you were made to feel guilty for not eating all your food ("Clean your plate—don't you know people are starving in Ethiopia!"), you'll likely believe that the amount of food on your plate is the most relevant determinant in how much to eat.[36] Alternatively, if your parents used a certain food as a reward ("Eat your vegetables and then you can have dessert!"), there's a good chance you'll think of that food in a negative context.[37] These and other psychological cues create nutritional beliefs that often stay with you into adulthood.

During adolescence, outside influences come into play with respect to nutrition.[38] The desire to "fit in" predominates during this period, increasing the likelihood of succumbing to peer pressures. Think back to your own adolescence. If all your friends were out eating pizza or cheeseburgers, you probably had a strong inclination to join in the fun; if they went to an arcade instead of playing sports, chances are you went along too. And given the fact that fast-food restaurants are now on almost every street corner and home video games are about as commonplace as TV sets, it's no wonder that the rate of teenage obesity has increased dramatically in recent times.

The contribution of sociologic factors on diet is generally greatest as an adult. It has been shown that episodes of overeating and impulsive eating are associated with such diverse situational circumstances as snacking alone, eating in the car, dining with friends, going to restaurants, having access to unhealthy foods, craving sweets, skipping meals, and being tired, irritable, bored, and/or depressed.[39] The take-home message is clear: To a great extent, you are a product of your environment.

The Pima Indians present an excellent case study on the contribution of environment on body weight. These Native Americans lived for centuries in the foothills of Arizona, leading an active lifestyle founded on hunting, fishing, and farming. This lifestyle persisted until the late 1800s, when their water supply was diverted by American settlers pushing westward. After suffering through a period of severe poverty and malnutrition, they were forced to survive on the typical high-fat, highly processed Western diet provided them by the United States government. Today, Arizona Pimas have the dubious distinction of having the highest rate of obesity and diabetes in the world.[40]

The plight of these Native Americans can be contrasted with a group of Pimas living in a remote, mountainous region of Mexico. Separated from their lineage about 1,000 years ago, the Mexican Pimas have the same genetic makeup as their Arizona counterparts. The difference, however, is that the Mexican Pimas continue to maintain a lifestyle consistent with that of their ancestors, working the fields to fend for food and eating a traditional diet.

As you may have guessed, the Mexican Pimas are a lot better off physically than the Pimas from Arizona. They have significantly less body fat and much lower incidences of diabetes and cardiovascular ailments—all despite a similar genetic predisposition to these abnormalities.[41,42] Moreover, when adjusted for percent of body fat, waist circumference, age, and sex, they also have higher circulating leptin levels[43]—a primary factor in successful long-term weight maintenance.

The good news is that it's easier to alter environmental factors than genetic factors. The human body is a very adaptive organism. Over time, it becomes accustomed to its environment and settles into a comfort zone. In fact, it's been hypothesized that any activity done consecutively for one month straight gets ingrained in your subconscious as routine. While acclimation might take a little longer for some than others, lifestyle changes will invariably develop into learned habits as long as they are implemented on a regular, consistent basis.

CHAPTER 3

The LGN Diet Solution

The information that follows is designed to help you overcome genetic and environmental obstacles, turning your body into a fat-burning machine. By teaching you how to eat the right combination of the right amounts of the right foods, you'll be able to attain a lean physique, one that looks great in or out of clothes. And you'll do all this safely, painlessly, and permanently, regardless of your present condition. Sound too good to be true? I can assure you it's not. Here's how the LGN program accomplishes these lofty objectives:

- *Regulates leptin:* As the master controller of set point, leptin is the most important hormone for long-term weight management. Hence, any successful fat-loss plan must exploit its utility. During dieting, however, this is easier said than done. Leptin production tends to drop sharply in times of caloric restriction (consistent with maintaining your set point) and most diets don't do anything to account for this untoward event. But while some reduction in leptin is inevitable as you lose weight, the LGN Diet keeps the drop to a minimum. And it works to improve leptin sensitivity, thereby increasing leptin transport into the brain. In this way, leptin is able to have a maximal impact on satiety and metabolism, overriding any attempt by your body to return to its set point.

- *Stabilizes blood glucose:* Secondary to leptin, blood glucose is a major determinant in regulating weight management. Wild swings in blood glucose are detrimental to body composition, both through a direct effect on the hypothalamus as well as by spiking the lipogenic hormone insulin. The LGN Diet is designed to stabilize blood glucose. By consuming unprocessed, nutrient-dense foods, you will maintain steady levels throughout the day. Not only does this aid in promoting satiety, but it also serves to keep the fat-storing effects of insulin at bay.

- *Diminishes hunger:* Hunger is one of the biggest obstacles to dietary adherence. The drive to eat is a powerful stimulus and, when left uncontrolled, binging is inevitable. This isn't a problem here. By focusing on foods with a high satiety value, the LGN Diet works to suppress appetite, with effects over and above those from the systems that regulate set point (i.e., leptin, blood glucose, etc.). You'll feel satisfied throughout the day, preventing the temptation to overindulge.

- *Preserves muscle:* If you want to optimize body composition, you need to maintain (or, better yet, increase) the amount of lean tissue that you carry. The trouble with most diets, however, is that they focus on weight loss without accounting for whether the reduction is in the form of fat or muscle. What a mistake! Losing muscle causes your metabolic rate to plummet, making weight regain inevitable—generally at levels higher than before. Not on the LGN Diet. Its emphasis on lean protein sources allows you to lose fat while holding on to your precious muscle tissue (or perhaps increasing it), and ensuring long-term sustainable results.

- *Enhances thermogenesis:* One of the ways your body expends energy is via a process called thermogenesis. Simply stated, thermogenesis is the dissipation of calories through the body's internal production of heat. The LGN Diet takes maximal advantage of the phenomenon. It incorporates foods and techniques that turn on various thermogenic processes, stoking your internal furnace and ratcheting up fat burning. This alone can result in the expenditure of a significant amount of calories per day.

- *Controls environment:* As stated, environmental factors account for about half of your diet-related results. The LGN Diet employs strategies that help you deal with your environment. Once you recognize the cues that trigger impulsive and/or unhealthy eating, you can take preventive actions to deal with these scenarios. Regardless of the setting or situation, you'll be in control of your environment—not vice versa—and have the where-withal to stay on the nutritional straight and narrow.

I realize I've put an awful lot of information on your plate so let me sum things up as simply as possible. Nature dealt you a certain body type. This body type is based on an individual set point that strives to maintain a given amount of fat. While most diets allow you to lose weight in the short term, they don't account for your set point, making weight regain inevitable. In contrast, the LGN Diet offers a permanent solution for changing your genetic disposition, allowing you to enjoy everlasting results.

By now you are undoubtedly excited by the prospect of redefining your physique. So without further ado, let's get into the meat and potatoes of the diet.

NUTRIENTS
FOR LIFE

PART TWO

CHAPTER 4

Curb Your Carbs

The LGN Diet has a number of key components that make it so successful, regardless of your present weight or "body type." Safe and scientifically sound, it allows you to regulate leptin, stabilize blood glucose, diminish hunger, preserve muscle, and enhance thermogenesis.

To accomplish these objectives, you need to have the right *amounts* of carbohydrates included in your daily meals and snacks. You also need to eat the right *kinds* of carbohydrates. These are the factors that I discuss in this chapter. Once you've adjusted your food intake so you're getting the right amounts and kinds of carbohydrates every day, you'll discover that long-term weight management becomes significantly easier to attain.

Before I make my recommendations, it needs to be acknowledged that there has been quite a lot of publicity, both pro and con, about the virtues of low carbohydrate (i.e., ketogenic) diets–the kind advocated by the late Dr. Robert Atkins and similar-minded "diet gurus." Many people have achieved substantial weight loss with these diets, but as you will see, there are several drawbacks inherent in the approach that make them detrimental to enduring dietary success.

In this chapter, you will find the guidelines you need to regulate and control your carbohydrate consumption for optimum benefits. I'll help you evaluate your body type, so you know what percentage of carbohydrates should be included in your daily meals. I'll discuss "nutrient density"—providing the guidelines you need to choose carbs that have a high concentration of vitamins, minerals, and fibers. You'll also learn some of the relative benefits of carbohydrates that come from vegetables as compared to those that come from fruit (which are high in natural sugars), and you'll discover some of the problems of refined sugar—that is, the kind that's found in candy, cakes, and other treats. There are, indeed, other ways to satisfy your sweet cravings!

TO CARB OR NOT TO CARB?

Now that you have an overview of where we're going, let's take care of some basics—specifically, what are carbohydrates? Simply stated, they are plant-based compounds that provide four calories of energy per gram. Think of them as circular links in a chain. A *monosaccharide* is a single link, a *disaccharide* is two links, and a *polysaccharide* is many links. In order to be utilized by the body, carbohydrates must be broken down into monosaccharides, of which there are three: glucose, fructose, and galactose. These monosaccharides are then used as an immediate source of energy or else stored for future use (either in the form of glycogen or fat).

Over the past few years, carbohydrates have gotten a bad rap. The recent low-carb craze has perpetuated the belief that all you have to do is eliminate carbohydrate intake and you'll magically lose weight. An entire industry has been spawned on this premise, with bestselling books and lines of low-carb supplements. Given the hype, millions of people are now avoiding carbs like they're the plague.

In truth, losing body fat is far more complex than simply eliminating carbs from your diet. There are many reasons why carbs, when eaten sensibly, can and should be an integral part of your nutritional regimen. To understand why, let's take a look at the science behind low-carb (i.e., ketogenic) diets.

Although every book on low-carb dieting has a slightly different wrinkle, they all share the same focus: inducing *ketosis*. Ketosis is a compensated state where the body shifts from using carbohydrates (glucose) to ketones—a by-product of the incomplete breakdown of fatty acids—for energy. Proponents of these diets profess that by regulating insulin function and shifting the body into a "fat-burning mode," ketosis optimizes weight loss while helping to preserve lean muscle tissue. With all the rhetoric, you'd think that ketogenic diets were a nutritional panacea. They're not.

Without question, low-carb diets help to stabilize insulin levels. Insulin is a storage hormone. While its primary purpose is to neutralize blood sugar, it also is responsible for shuttling fat into fat cells.[1] When carbohydrates are ingested, the pancreas secretes insulin to clear blood sugar from the circulatory system. Depending on the quantities and types of carbs consumed, insulin levels can fluctuate wildly, heightening the possibility of fat storage.[2]

Making matters worse, many people are insulin resistant—as much as a quarter of the population, by some estimates. It is postulated that anyone who is clinically obese (i.e., more than 20 percent over his or her ideal body weight) has at least some degree of insulin resistance. This condition obstructs glucose from entering target cells, resulting in the conversion of carbohydrate to fat (through a process called *lipogenesis*). A vicious cycle is created, whereby fat storage is increased and insulin resistance is heightened even further. Eventually, this can lead to the onset of non-insulin-dependent diabetes (NIDD)—a serious disease that can potentially cause blindness, stroke, and even death.

However, although low-carb diets are quite effective at regulating blood sugar, by no means are they necessary to combat insulin resistance. For the great majority of people, simply cutting back carb intake to more moderate levels is sufficient to accomplish this task.[3] Even in extreme cases, a drastic reduction in carbohydrates rarely is needed to stabilize insulin levels.

There is scant evidence that inducing a state of ketosis actually helps to accelerate fat loss and/or preserve muscle.[4] While the rationale behind a "fat-burning mode" sounds great in theory, it simply doesn't translate into practice. Studies have repeatedly shown that it's the total energy intake, rather than the composition of macronutrients, that is the major determinant in the loss of body fat.[5] This is consistent with a law of thermodynamics: if you expend more calories than you consume, you'll lose weight. Provided there is a caloric deficit, the body seems to adjust its nutrient utilization, burning similar amounts of fat regardless of dietary nutritional composition.

But what about all those testimonials from people claiming to have lost as much as fifteen pounds in the first two weeks of low-carb dieting? Well, much of this reduction is due to a loss of fluids—not body fat.[6] You see, carbs have a propensity to attract water in the body (each gram of stored carbohydrate draws in about three times its weight in water). So when carbs are removed from the diet, diuresis is encouraged, causing the kidneys to excrete water. While this can provide a psychological boost in the early stages of dieting, the carryover doesn't last long. As soon as the diet is discontinued and carbs are reintroduced into your system, all of the water weight returns—an outcome that can be extremely disheartening (and even cause post-diet depression).

The real "magic" behind low-carb diets is their effect on appetite suppression; when carbs are restricted, food cravings tend to subside. Although the exact mechanisms are somewhat unclear, it's theorized that increased secretions of satiety hormones play an integral role in the process. The hormones cholecystokinin (CCK) and glucagon, in particular, have been shown to quell hunger sensations, reducing the urge to eat.[7]

Additionally, due to a limited number of food choices, there is less pleasure associated with eating low-carb meals. With reduced variety, a diet becomes mundane. After several months of subsisting on nothing but protein and fat, most people never want to look at another piece of steak or cheese again. The net result: a diminished caloric intake.[8,9] This is the philosophy behind the assertions of various low-carb gurus that you can eat as much as you want on this type of diet; they know you won't!

Although the associated health risks have been largely overblown (there is no evidence ketosis causes liver or kidney damage in healthy people), several things make these diets undesirable for long-term use.

First, ketogenic diets can have an adverse effect on mood.[10] Remember that ketosis is a compensated state, outside the realm of "normal" bodily function. Since the brain runs on a steady supply of glucose, it is particularly sensitive to a deficiency. When carbs are restricted, the brain is forced to adjust to using ketones as an alternate energy source. The adjustment to ketone utilization takes several weeks, and, during this time, people invariably become lethargic and weak. Mental acuity is compromised, making it difficult to concentrate on complex tasks. All in all, the transition period is usually most unpleasant. And while some seem to regain their energy levels once adaptation has taken place, others don't. It is not uncommon for low-carb dieters to complain they are walking around in a constant state of malaise, feeling sluggish and physically drained throughout the day.

Another side effect of low-carb diets is that they cause halitosis (bad breath). During ketosis, there is a buildup of acetone (one of the primary ketone bodies), which is then excreted from the body both in the urine and via respiration. The problem is, acetone has a funky odor (it is the ingredient that gives nail polish remover its distinct smell). After a while, your breath ends up smelling like a nail salon during busy season. And rest assured, it doesn't matter how good you look if nobody wants to come within five feet of you!

In addition, ketogenic diets have a negative effect on leptin. They reduce leptin production and, depending on the types of fats consumed, can actually contribute to leptin resistance.[11,12] Hypothetically, this can raise your set point, making it increasingly difficult to stay lean over the long term.

Ketogenic diets also are detrimental to exercise performance (I discuss in Chapter 10 why exercise is so essential to long-term weight management).[13,14] The compounds derived from carbohydrate breakdown are stored as glycogen in your muscles and liver. Glycogen is the primary fuel used to power your muscles during intense workouts. It provides an instant source of energy that can be accessed on demand, enabling you to work out intensely. When glycogen stores are depleted (as happens when you go into ketosis), your body has to convert amino acids into glucose (through a process called gluconeogenesis) in order to meet short-term energy needs. However, this conversion process is very inefficient and fails to supply adequate fuel for training. Within a short period of time, your stamina begins to wane and you ultimately "run out of gas."

Moreover, the very low insulin levels associated with ketosis are an impediment to gaining muscle. Contrary to popular belief, insulin isn't just an "evil" hormone whose sole purpose is to promote fat storage. When properly regulated, it plays a central role in building lean tissue. Specifically, insulin is both anabolic (helping to manufacture body proteins) and anti-catabolic (helping to prevent the breakdown of body proteins).[15,16] The bottom line: without carbs, muscle development suffers.

Perhaps the biggest problem associated with low-carb diets is that the vast majority of people can't (and, for health reasons, probably shouldn't) stick with them over the long haul. Adherence is the most important aspect of any nutritional program, and, with so little variety, low-carb diets simply are too restrictive to sustain. Once you go off the regimen, the question then becomes, "Now what?" Most people simply aren't prepared to return to a balanced diet. They don't know how to eat properly and, in the absence of a structured plan, are apt to gain back everything they lost.

HOW MUCH IS TOO MUCH?

Taking all factors into consideration, carbohydrates should be an important component of any nutritional regimen that seeks to optimize body composition. Now, this is not to imply that a diet very high in carbs is desirable for these purposes. It's not. Except for perhaps ultra-endurance athletes, carbohydrate intake in excess of 60 percent of total calories is counterproductive. For most, it only serves to exacerbate blood sugar levels, increase triglycerides, and cause unwanted fat deposition.

The key is to consume the right amount of carbohydrate for your body: enough to keep your body running at peak efficiency, but not too much so as to spike blood glucose and insulin levels. This is where many diets fail. There is no standardized formula that works for everyone. Carbohydrate sensitivity varies from person to person, and, in order to optimize results, an individualized prescription is required.

DISCOVERING YOUR BODY TYPE

So how do you go about determining your ideal carb ratio? Glad you asked. Based on a wealth of research and personal experience, I have discovered that the best way to estimate carbohydrate intake is by body type. In the 1940s, William H. Sheldon developed a general classification system for identifying a person by body structure called somatotyping, and identified three body types called ectomorph, mesomorph, and endomorph. Incorporating his body structure typing with the concept of the set point, I have defined three distinct body types:

- *Type I:* Type I individuals are usually large framed. They are big and soft, with a propensity to hoard body fat. Prime examples include football linemen and voluptuous pinup girls. If you have difficulty getting lean, you are probably Type I. Because of increased fat deposits, people who are Type I have a predisposition toward insulin resistance.[17] Hence, they tend to do best with a lower carb intake, in the range of about 35 to 40 percent of total calories. This helps to control blood glucose levels while supplying the body with enough carbs to fuel metabolic needs.
- *Type II:* Type II individuals tend to be muscular with fairly low levels of body fat. They have athletic physiques and typically have few problems gaining or losing weight. This is the classic bodybuilding structure and often is seen in sprinters, swimmers, and fitness models. Type IIs generally function well on a moderate carbohydrate protocol, consuming 45 to 50 percent of calories from carbs.
- *Type III:* Type III individuals are lean and lanky, with low amounts of fat and muscle. They are notorious "hardgainers," finding it difficult to increase muscularity. Think of marathon runners and runway models as examples of this body type. Type IIIs generally excel on a higher carb intake, in the range of 55 to 60 percent of total calories. This helps to maximize anabolic (tissue-building) function without having a significant impact on fat accumulation.

It should be noted that rarely do you find people who are "pure" Type I, Type II, or Type III. Rather, they are amalgams of each type, with qualities that lie somewhere between two of the classifications. With this in mind, take a look at your physique in a mirror. Where do you fit in on the continuum? If you tend to

> ## Percent of Calories from Carbohydrates, Based on Body Type
>
> Type I: 35 to 40 percent
> Type II: 45 to 50 percent
> Type III: 55 to 60 percent

store fat easily, you'd probably do best with the lower carb intake associated with a Type I. On the other hand, if you are someone who has trouble gaining weight, the higher carb intake associated with a Type III would likely be most appropriate. If you are somewhere in the middle, opt for the moderate carb intake associated with a Type II. It's that easy! You now have a handle on the approximate amount of carbs to include in your diet.

Realize, though, that while body typing provides a sensible method for estimating ideal carb intake, it is by no means absolute. Other factors, both genetic and environmental, can influence carbohydrate sensitivity. Hence, use these guidelines as a starting point. See how your body responds to a given carb ratio and, if you don't see the desired results after a fair period of time, make adjustments as needed. (Specific guidelines will be given in Chapter 8.)

A COMPLEX QUANDARY: UNDERSTANDING CARBOHYDRATES

Now that we've covered carbohydrate quantity, let's turn our attention to qualitative issues. Standard nutritional advice has always been to eat "complex" carbs and avoid "simple" carbs. This is based on the belief that simple carbs have a negative effect on insulin (they are hyperinsulemic) while complex carbs are "insulin friendly." Given the detriments associated with an oversecretion of insulin, the preference for complex carbs certainly seems justified.

The truth is, however, carbohydrates don't always behave according to their complexity. For instance, it has been determined that many complex carbs like potatoes and white bread actually cause a large insulin response while simple carbs such as apples and oranges don't.[18,19] This turns the whole complex carb theory on its head.

The Glycemic Index

In an attempt to understand carbohydrates, some have suggested to choose carbs by their rating on the glycemic index. Originally created to help diabetics adjust their insulin dosage, the glycemic index ranks foods on how they affect blood sugar levels. By measuring the speed at which carbs enter the bloodstream, it provides a reasonably accurate indication of their impact on insulin secretion.[20] Carbs that cause a rapid elevation of blood sugar (i.e., glucose) are termed high glycemic, while those that are "timed-release" and maintain stable levels of blood sugar are called low glycemic.

Due to their effect on insulin levels, high-glycemic carbs tend to be *lipogenic* (i.e., fat-promoting).[21,22] Remember, insulin is a storage hormone that turns on various fat-storage mechanisms and blocks certain enzymes that are responsible for fat breakdown. When insulin levels are high, excess nutrients are more readily shuttled into fat cells, resulting in an increase in body fat. Not a desirable scenario for someone trying to stay lean.

Furthermore, high insulin levels can also create a vicious cycle that encourages binge eating.[23] A rush of insulin clears sugars from your circulatory system so quickly that it creates a rebound effect, producing a sudden and dramatic drop in blood sugar levels. A hypoglycemic state is induced, causing severe hunger pangs and food cravings. As a result, more calories are consumed (especially in the form of high-glycemic foods) and fat storage is heightened even further.

Low-glycemic foods, on the other hand, are processed slowly. They enter the bloodstream in a timed-release fashion, keeping blood sugar levels in check.[24] As a result, insulin is stabilized, reducing the potential for unwanted fat accumulation.

But while the glycemic index is a nifty tool for evaluating carbohydrates, it has several shortcomings. For one, food isn't consumed in a vacuum. A meal generally consists of a combination of different foods: spaghetti with meatballs, rice with chicken, etc. When fats and proteins are consumed with a carbohydrate, digestion is slowed and the glycemic response is mitigated. Thus, under most conditions, the glycemic index is of limited utility.

More important, the glycemic index fails to distinguish whether or not a food has nutritional value. For instance, a carrot has a higher glycemic score than a Snickers bar. Now which do you think is more nutritious? The carrot, of course. Numerous other items such as doughnuts and ice cream also have low ratings, yet by no means could they be classified as "healthy" foods. All things considered, it is imprudent to solely rely on the glycemic index to guide your choice of carbohydrate.

The Importance of Nutrient Density

Fortunately, there is a better yardstick for assessing which carbohydrates to eat and which to avoid: nutrient density. Nutrient density takes into account the amount of vitamins and minerals (discussed in Chapter 13) as well as fiber (discussed later in this chapter) in a carbohydrate. Not only are nutrient-dense carbs insulin friendly, but they also supply your body with essential compounds that enhance metabolic function.[25,26] Many of the vitamins and minerals are used as coenzymes that assist the body in fat burning. Others serve as antioxidants that keep cells functioning optimally. And fiber promotes satiety, decreasing the urge to overeat.

In contrast, non-nutrient-dense foods are empty calories. The worst offenders are processed (refined) carbs. They contribute little to bodily processes and send blood sugar levels sky-high. Making matters worse, the excessive consumption of these foods can directly lead to insulin resistance.[27] By stimulating large amounts of insulin on a repeated basis, glucose receptors are forced to work overtime. Eventually, receptors become desensitized to insulin (an anomaly known as *downregulation*) and glucose cannot be stored as efficiently.[28] The net result: increased fat storage.[29,30]

THE BIG THREE CARBOHYDRATES

There are three main types of carbohydrate-based foods: grains, fruits, and vegetables. I will discuss each of them individually and explain how they should best be incorporated into your diet.

Grains

Grains are long chains of glucose strung together (called a starch). The digestion of starch begins almost as soon as it enters your mouth when an enzyme called *salivary amylase* begins to degrade the glucose chain. Digestion continues through the gastrointestinal tract until the starch eventually is converted into single "links" of

---

The Dough Ball Test

Many of the whole-wheat sandwich breads sold in stores are merely bran-fortified and are therefore not much better than their white counterparts. Good breads are very coarse and grainy rather than soft and squishy. A reliable method for analysis is the Dough Ball Test: If the bread can be rolled into a compact ball, it's a poor choice; if it breaks into pieces, it's a keeper.

---

glucose and absorbed through the intestinal wall. Examples of starches include bread, rice, and pasta—popular staples in the American diet.

There is a growing sentiment, however, that starches are the root of nutritional evil. Some "experts" even go so far as to claim that the only way to lose weight is by cutting out all starches from the diet. The supposed problem has to do with the fact that they are composed of glucose. Once glucose traverses the intestinal wall, it bypasses liver metabolism and goes directly into circulation. If this happens in a rapid fashion, blood sugar levels skyrocket, insulin levels spike, and there is an increased chance of unwanted fat deposition.

Realize, though, that not all starches are alike. It's the ones made from refined grains and white flour that send insulin through the roof and switch on the mechanisms that promote fat accumulation. Accordingly, stay away from white pasta, white rice, white flour breads, sweetened cereals, and other processed starches. Instead, adhere to the slogan "Think brown," and consume nutrient-dense alternatives such as whole-wheat pasta, brown rice, oatmeal, and multigrain bread. Brown carbs are "slow

---

Celiac Disease

Approximately 1 in every 200 people suffers from celiac disease, also known as gluten intolerance. This condition results from an autoimmune response to the ingestion of gluten, a protein found in various grain sources. Symptoms include bloating, diarrhea, muscle cramps, and weakness. If you are afflicted, you must refrain from eating wheat, rye, and barley and derivatives of these grains.

---

burning," ensuring that glucose enters circulation in a timed-release fashion. Ultimately, insulin remains stable and the potential for fat storage is diminished.

Finally, what often goes overlooked is the fact that starches provide a concentrated source of calories. An ounce of pasta, for example, contains about 100 calories while an ounce of lean protein contains less than one-third of that amount. So watch your portions carefully. A small mistake in estimating quantity can add up to a lot of extra calories. Nutrient density notwithstanding, overconsumption is the primary reason why starches tend to pack on the pounds.

Fruit

Fruits are a unique breed of carbohydrate. They contain large amounts of a sugar called fructose. Unlike glucose, which bypasses the liver and goes directly into the bloodstream, fructose is metabolized by the liver. Since the liver slows absorption into the circulatory system, blood glucose and insulin remain more stable when fructose is consumed. Hence, fruits tend to have a low glycemic rating. Combined with the fact that they are replete in vitamins, minerals, and fiber, fruits would seem to be an ideal carbohydrate for weight loss. But lo and behold, this doesn't always translate into practice.

To appreciate why, a little physiology is necessary. Only two bodily tissues can store carbohydrate in the form of glycogen: the muscles and the liver. Depending on body type, the liver has the ability to store about 50 grams per day (approximately 200 calories' worth) while the muscles can store more than five times this amount (approximately 1,000 calories' worth). Muscles, however, lack an enzyme that converts fructose into glycogen. Thus, while glucose-based carbohydrates (such as starches) can be stored in both muscle and liver tissue, fructose is almost exclusively stored in the liver. And herein lies the problem. Once liver glycogen is full, the body starts converting fructose into triglycerides—the precursors of body fat. Thus, an excess intake of fructose is more likely to result in fat deposition when compared with other forms of carbohydrate.[31,32]

Despite this drawback, fruits are a quality carb source. They are nutrient dense and supply healthy amounts of antioxidants that are difficult to get from other foods (see Chapter 13 for a discussion of antioxidants). Moreover, their sweet taste can help to satisfy sugar cravings, thereby reducing the intake of cakes and candies. The key is to monitor consumption. A good rule of thumb is to limit daily intake to three to four medium-sized pieces of fruit. Be especially careful with dried fruits such as raisins and prunes. When a fruit is dehydrated, it isn't as filling (water helps to promote satiety) and consequently tends to promote overeating.

The Juicing Myth

Don't believe the hype that fruit juice is healthier than whole fruits. Juicing removes fiber from a fruit as well as some of its vitamins and minerals. This of course reduces a fruit's nutrient density, rendering it less beneficial.

In addition, since liquids require very little digestion, they quickly pass through your gastrointestinal tract and are rapidly assimilated. This not only increases blood sugar and insulin levels, but it also has less of an effect on satiety. So, despite the claims of various "juicer" infomercials, fruit juice is a poor substitute for whole fruits except when used as a post-exercise drink (see Chapter 10 for specific information on nutrition as it relates to exercise).

Vegetables

Vegetables are among the most nutrient-dense foods in the world. In addition to being rich in vitamins, minerals, and fiber, they also contain substances called phytochemicals. Phytochemicals, which go by such obscure names as indoles and isothiocyanates, are rapidly becoming one of the most exciting areas in the field of nutrition. Research is still emerging, but they have already been shown to provide numerous health-related benefits, and are believed to have anti-aging properties. As scientists conduct further studies, phytochemicals may very well turn out to be the closest thing to a nutritional fountain of youth.

Of all the different kinds of vegetables, greens are at the top of the list. Think of them as green water, "freebies" that can be consumed in large amounts without making you fat. A pound of broccoli, for instance, contains only about 120 calories (compare that with a pound of pasta, which has about 1,600 calories!). Spinach, kale, collard greens, asparagus, and Brussels sprouts are equally low in calories and high in nutritional value. A notable exception is peas, which contain higher concentrations of starch and therefore should be eaten in moderation.

Salads are always a good choice for dieters. As a rule, opt for the darker-colored leaves. They are more nutrient dense, with much greater concentrations of vitamins and minerals. So ditch the iceberg lettuce; arugula and romaine are better alternatives.

Certain other veggies require more dietary scrutiny. Winter squash and carrots have about double the amount of calories as green vegetables so pay attention to intake when eating these foods. And while corn and potatoes (including yams) are technically vegetables, they actually behave like starches and, in the context of your diet, should be considered in the same category as rice or pasta.

THE FIBER FACTOR

Fiber is the Rodney Dangerfield of nutrients: it doesn't get any respect. While carbs, protein, or fat are at the forefront of every nutritional discussion, fiber is often relegated to second-tier status. But make no mistake, fiber has many functions that are vital to your body. A deficiency is bound to cause problems.

Fiber is made up of several different components, including cellulose, lignin, pectins, mucilages, and other plant-based materials, each with their own distinctive dietary properties. It is unique in that it cannot be completely digested (due to the fact that the body lacks an enzyme called *cellulase,* which is responsible for breaking down fiber in the gastrointestinal system) and therefore passes into the colon unimpeded. Since fiber has virtually no caloric value, its consumption can't make you gain weight!

There is a large body of scientific evidence indicating that a diet high in fiber is beneficial to your health. For one, it helps to maintain bowel regularity. Because it soaks up bodily fluids like a sponge, fiber makes your stools soft and fluffy, preventing constipation. The increase in stool volume also helps to dilute the concentration of bile acids, which are thought to instigate the growth of malignant tumors. Research seems to back up this hypothesis: studies have shown that modest increases in fiber consumption reduce the risk of colorectal cancer by more than 30 percent![33]

In addition, fiber consumption can cause a substantial decline in serum cholesterol levels. Reductions of up to 18 percent have been reported, with favorable effects on the ratio of "good" to "bad" cholesterol (HDL to LDL).[34] Since each 1 percent drop in cholesterol translates into a 2 percent drop in the risk of developing heart disease, the cardioprotective effects of fiber are far reaching.

Fiber also helps to support colonic bacteria. These bacteria, called microflora, are detoxifiers. They scavenge your body, ridding it of various contaminants. When fiber enters the colon, some of it ferments into short-chain fatty acids, a valuable source of fuel. Microflora feast on the short-chain fatty acids, giving them the energy to carry out their regulatory functions.

Besides having a positive effect on your well-being, fiber also plays an important role in weight management.[35] By forming a viscous "gel" in the intestines, fiber delays gastric emptying, causing nutrients to stay in the stomach longer. This has dual benefits. First, blood sugar levels stabilize as carbohydrates are gradually assimilated into circulation, allowing your body to utilize them on a slow, steady basis. Second, hunger is suppressed. The stomach has "stretch sensors" that regulate food intake. When food builds up in the stomach, a satiety signal is sent to the brain and you feel satisfied. Fiber is so good at filling you up that a mere 14 gram increase has been shown to result in a 10 percent reduction in energy intake.[36]

What's more, the fibrous "gel" actually inhibits the digestion and absorption of nutrients. As food passes through your gastrointestinal tract, some of the nutrients get trapped in the gel and end up being excreted before they can be metabolized. This is especially true of fats, which, when bound to fiber, cannot pass through the intestinal wall. The net result is that you can eat more food without having it stored in your system. In fact, it has been reported that, by simply doubling fiber intake from 18 to 36 grams, you reduce the calories in your diet by more than 100 calories per day![37]

Fiber is found in a wide array of plant-based foods, especially unrefined grains, fruits, and vegetables. Table 4.1 shows some of the more popular high-fiber foods as well as their corresponding fiber content. Consume them readily. By maintaining a high-fiber diet, you'll go a long way to improving your health as well as your body.

Table 4.1

HIGH-FIBER FOODS		
FOOD	**AMOUNT**	**FIBER CONTENT (g)**
Apple	1 medium	3
All-bran cereal	1 ounce	10
Barley	1 cup	6
Blackberries	1 cup	8
Black beans	1 cup	19
Blueberries	1 cup	4
Bread (whole-wheat)	2 slices	6
Broccoli	1 cup	8

FOOD	AMOUNT	FIBER CONTENT (g)
Brussels sprouts	1 cup	7
Chickpeas	1 cup	12
Corn	1 medium	5
Grape-Nuts cereal	1 cup	7
Green peas	1 cup	18
Kidney beans	1 cup	11
Lentils	1 cup	15
Oatmeal	½ cup	4
Pear	1 medium	4
Pinto beans	1 cup	15
Raspberries	1 cup	9
Rice (brown)	½ cup	5
Soybeans	1 cup	10
Spinach	1 cup	7
Yam	1 medium	7

Fiber intake should exceed 20 grams per 1,000 calories consumed, with a minimum of about 30 grams per day. In most cases, this is easily achieved by eating a variety of nutrient-dense carbohydrates. If your total caloric intake falls below about 1,500 calories a day, however, it's possible that you won't get enough fiber from whole foods. In this case, consider taking one of the many fiber supplements on the market. They are quick and convenient, allowing you to fiber up without a great deal of hassle.

There is a point of diminishing returns with fiber, though. Excess intake, above about 60 grams a day, can interfere with the metabolism of various minerals, particularly calcium, zinc, and iron. So, while it's great to fiber up, don't go too far overboard.

WHAT ABOUT SWEETS?

Sweets are the downfall of many a dieter. Even the most steadfast dieters can't resist the allure of cookies, cakes, and candies (not to mention soft drinks such as colas, lemonades, and iced teas). The temptation is simply too much to bear.

Contributing to their popularity is the fact that sweets are addicting. For both psychological as well as physiological reasons, sugar makes you crave more sugar. Have a piece of chocolate cake and you want another . . . then another . . . and another. Before you know it, you've polished off half the cake. No matter how much you eat, you're never satisfied.

The primary ingredient in most sweets is sucrose, which contains equal amounts of glucose and fructose. Sucrose, also known as table sugar, is an "empty calorie" with no nutritional value. While most people have been led to believe it's important to cut back on dietary fat, they often are oblivious to the detriments of refined sugar. The fact is that sweets can be as bad as, or even worse than, greasy, fried cuisine.

The main problem with sucrose is its high fructose content. As previously discussed, your body has a limited capacity to store fructose. Once daily consumption exceeds about 50 grams, the body begins converting fructose into triglycerides for storage as body fat. Since sweets have addictive qualities that tend to promote excess consumption (as opposed to fruits, which, because of their fibrous nature, have a satiating effect), they bombard your system with fructose and invariably have a negative effect on body composition.

Even worse, many sweets contain an additive called high-fructose corn syrup (HFCS). Because it is cheaper than sucrose, HFCS has made its way into thousands of products, including carbonated beverages, baked goods, canned fruits, jams and jellies, and dairy products. Why is HFCS so bad? Well, while sucrose contains about 50 percent fructose, HFCS can contain upward of 90 percent. Considering what you now know about fructose and its effect on the body, the detriments of HFCS should be obvious.

All things considered, the best advice is to avoid sweets as much as possible, especially those that contain HFCS. In order to avoid hidden sources, learn to read labels. Stay away from any product that has sucrose or high-fructose corn syrup (also listed as "natural fruit sweeteners") listed as one of the first few ingredients.

Finding Hidden Sugars: How to Read Food Labels

In order to avoid hidden sugars in foods, carefully read food labels to look for the following names for refined sugars:

- *HFCS:* High-fructose corn syrup
- *Natural Fruit Sweeteners:* High-fructose corn syrup

You'll never eliminate all refined sugars from your diet, but, with a little effort and discipline, you certainly can keep their intake to a minimum.

Many people, however, simply can't do without having something sweet in their diet. Women, in particular, have a tendency to be "sweetaholics." This is largely due to hormonal fluctuations associated with the menstrual cycle. During menstruation, serotonin levels in the brain drop precipitously. Serotonin is a neurotransmitter that helps to regulate mood, and the lower levels that are often associated with menstruation can result in a depressive state. Well it just so happens that carbs, especially simple sugars, help to raise serotonin production.[38] So women have a physiologic drive to eat sweets during this period—by elevating serotonin levels, it makes them feel better.

Fortunately, there are several things you can do to satisfy your sweet tooth without binging on junk food. One of the best options is to eat fruit. As long as you keep consumption to three to four medium pieces a day, fruit is a nutritional home run. Kiwis, watermelon, papaya, and various berries are among the sweetest-tasting fruits and make excellent choices as a snack or dessert.

Another option is to consume products that use a sugar substitute such as aspartame (commonly known as NutraSweet). Aspartame is 200 times as sweet as sucrose and therefore only minute quantities are required to achieve desired effects. Basically, sweetening a product with aspartame enhances flavor without adding calories—a definite win/win situation. Moreover, as opposed to sugar-based foods, aspartame doesn't increase appetite; in fact, it actually helps to suppress it.[39] Studies have shown that simply switching from foods sweetened with sugar to those sweetened with aspartame can significantly reduce caloric consumption.[40] The implications are clear: Aspartame can facilitate the loss of body fat and contribute to long-term weight maintenance.

Inexplicably, various factions have sprung up espousing the theory that aspartame is responsible for conditions as diverse as multiple sclerosis, Alzheimer's dis-

---

Tips to Satisfy Your Sweet Tooth

- Eat sweet fruits (no more than 4 medium pieces a day), particularly kiwis, watermelon, papaya, and berries.
- Use or eat foods that contain sugar substitutes such as NutraSweet and Splenda.
- Chew sugar-free gum.
- Eat frozen yogurt.
- Suck on sugar-free candy.
- Drink diet soda.

---

ease, Parkinson's disease, diabetes, Gulf War syndrome, and brain tumors. Entire Web sites have been established to champion the "ban aspartame" cause. There are even aspartame support groups aimed at helping people who have suffered from so-called "aspartame poisoning." All of this hoopla has created an alarmist mentality, striking fear among the general public.

A review of the facts, however, shows that aspartame has been unfairly maligned. Before its approval in the early 1980s, the United States Food and Drug Administration (FDA) studied aspartame more thoroughly than any other food additive in history.[41] To date, more than 500 peer-reviewed research studies have been performed on the supplement. Yet, by all accounts, there is no evidence whatsoever that it is harmful in otherwise healthy individuals.[42]

Technically, aspartame does have the potential to negatively affect brain function. It is derived from the amino acid phenylalanine (as well as aspartic acid), which in extremely high concentrations can be neurotoxic. As seen in the disease phenylketonuria (PKU), the uptake of massive quantities of phenylalanine by the brain results in a variety of psychological disorders, including memory loss, seizures, and, in extreme cases, mental retardation.

In reality, though, it's virtually impossible to consume enough aspartame to bring about neurotoxic effects. You'd have to drink approximately 50 liters of diet soda a day in order to reach the threshold for toxicity! But the average consumer never even approaches the upper limits of what is deemed to be an acceptable daily intake (ADI) by the FDA.[43] Since "acceptable" levels are considered to be a "safe" range, the potential for someone to develop serious side effects as a result of aspartame consumption is virtually nonexistent.

The supposed link between aspartame and cancer is also unsubstantiated.[44]

Upon ingestion, aspartame is processed in the gastrointestinal tract and broken down into its constituent amino acids, aspartic acid and phenylalanine.[45] Neither aspartame nor its components accumulate in the body over time. Given that these same amino acids are present in large amounts in meats, beans, and dairy products, and are assimilated in the exact same fashion, it therefore follows that aspartame is no more carcinogenic than any other food source.

Some people do claim to experience minor adverse reactions from aspartame, even at fairly low levels of intake. This most probably is related to its influence on tryptophan—an amino acid that's a precursor for the brain chemical serotonin. Tryptophan and phenylalanine are antagonistic; they compete with each other to cross the blood-brain barrier. If the concentration of phenylalanine is substantially higher than that of tryptophan, serotonin levels can fall precipitously. Occasionally, this can exacerbate various mood disorders and those with clinical depression are somewhat vulnerable.[46] But this is of no long-term consequence: if symptoms arise, simply discontinue use and any negative complications will quickly subside.

There are several other artificial sweeteners on the market that are viable alternatives to aspartame. Of note is sucralose (marketed under the name Splenda). Su-

Summary of the Look Great Naked Diet Guidelines for Carbohydrate

1. Estimate the percentage of carbohydrate in your diet by body type: Type Is should consume about 35 to 40 percent carbs, Type IIs should consume about 45 to 50 percent carbs, and Type IIIs should consume about 55 to 60 percent carbs.

2. Evaluate carbs by their nutrient density. Those that have ample amounts of vitamins, minerals, and fiber should be chosen over those that don't.

3. With respect to grains, remember the phrase "Think brown." Eliminate refined carbohydrates from your diet and replace them with whole grains.

4. Eat fruit but limit intake to 3 to 4 medium-sized pieces per day. Choose whole fruits over juices.

5. Load up on vegetables. Consume greens at will, but consume high-starch vegetables moderately.

6. Keep your consumption of sweets to a minimum and avoid products that contain high-fructose corn syrup. Artificial sweeteners can be used to satisfy sugar cravings.

cralose is a derivative of sucrose. Since for the most part it can't be digested by the body, it has no effect on caloric intake. And like aspartame, it has been well researched (more than 100 peer-reviewed studies) and met with FDA approval.

Sucralose has a distinct benefit over aspartame in that it can withstand high heat and therefore can be used in cooking. Some people also claim it has less of an aftertaste than aspartame, but this, of course, is subjective. The best advice is to try both and see which one you prefer.

CHAPTER 5

The Power of Protein

Balance is important in all things in life—and it's absolutely essential in nutrition. Just as I do not endorse low-carb diets, I wouldn't recommend an ultra-high-carb diet either, at least as a long-term strategy. To get the most from your body, your intake of carbohydrate and proteins needs to be balanced.

The LGN Diet introduces a very easy way to do this "balancing act." By following a simple set of guidelines, you'll be able to calculate how much protein you should be getting every day. But before I make those recommendations, I think it's important to understand the key role that protein plays in contributing to your energy and overall health.

The amount and the kind of protein in your diet affects many factors related to critical body mechanisms. Every aspect of your body is influenced by protein—including your muscle and skin tone, bone density, and metabolism. The amount of protein in your diet will have an impact on how hungry you feel, primarily because it affects hormones that suppress appetite. It also has an impact on insulin levels, modulating the way that sugars are absorbed by your body. In this chapter, I will describe exactly how these mechanisms work.

For many years, the U.S. Department of Agriculture has published Recommended Dietary Allowance (RDA) guidelines that specify how much protein should be in our diets. In order to optimize body composition, I advocate a protein intake *higher* than what is specified by the RDA. This additional protein can come from a wide variety of lean sources—fish, beef, and dairy, as well as certain grains and legumes (including soy)—so you'll have optimum levels for good health and energy. High-quality protein powders can be beneficial if you know how and when to take advantage of them. There's a lot of ground to cover but all of these issues and more will be explored in detail.

THE ANABOLIC ADVANTAGE

Every cell in your body contains protein. Your skin, hair, nails, internal organs, muscles, and even bones utilize protein to various extents in their development. Pure and simple, protein is the king of all nutrients: life could not go on without it.

From a biochemical perspective, proteins are linked chains of amino acids called polypeptides. Amino acids are divided into two basic categories: essential and nonessential. The essential amino acids (leucine, tryptophan, lysine, methionine, phenylalanine, threonine, valine, histidine, and isoleucine) are the most nutritionally significant. These amino acids cannot be manufactured by the body and therefore must be obtained from the foods in your diet. A deficiency in any one can have dire consequences.

In order to maintain their integrity and adapt to environmental stresses, your cells undergo constant *remodeling,* using amino acids as the raw materials for repair. Some tissues such as the liver remodel in a matter of hours while others such as tendons and ligaments can take months before turnover is fully completed. Muscle, which makes up the majority of lean body tissue, remodels over a period of several days.

During remodeling, your body operates like a factory, continuously breaking down old proteins (called *catabolism*) and building new ones (called *anabolism*). While some of the degraded proteins are reused, others are burned for energy or excreted in the feces, sweat, and other bodily processes. This constitutes the body's net protein losses.

The only way to replenish lost proteins is by consuming foods that contain protein. Here is a simplified version of how it works: After ingestion, protein enters the stomach where it is partially broken down into smaller polypeptides by hydrochloric acid and the enzyme pepsin. The polypeptides empty into the small intestine where they are further divided into a combination of single amino acids, *dipeptides* (two amino acids bound together) and *tripeptides* (three amino acids bound together). Anything larger than a tripeptide is not well absorbed through the intestinal wall and must undergo further breakdown. Once in the bloodstream, amino acids are then transported to various tissues to assist in repair and growth.

Protein status in the body is determined by nitrogen balance: A negative nitrogen balance means your body is breaking down proteins at a greater rate than it's synthesizing them; a positive nitrogen balance means your body is creating new proteins faster than it is breaking them down; and a stable nitrogen balance means protein degradation and protein synthesis are in equilibrium.

Based on this information, it should be obvious that a protein-rich diet is essential for optimizing body composition. If your intake of protein is insufficient to make up for what is excreted, cellular function is compromised and your appearance, as well as overall health, suffers. Only by consuming protein in excess of losses can you promote anabolism and enhance the quality of your physique.

THE METABOLIC EDGE

In addition to its anabolic role, protein also has unique metabolic actions. A large percentage of calories from protein are burned off in the digestion process—a phenomenon called the *thermic effect of food* (TEF). Of all the macronutrients, protein has the highest thermic effect, burning off approximately 25 percent of the calories consumed. In comparison, only 10 percent of the calories from carbs are burned off in digestion; fat has virtually no thermic effect whatsoever.[1] When the TEF is factored into a mixed meal, higher intakes of protein can as much as double postprandial thermogenesis (i.e., the number of calories burned after eating), leaving fewer calories available to be stored as fat.

Further, protein tends to curb appetite.[2,3] During its digestion, protein promotes the secretion of a hormone called cholecystokinin (CCK), which acts to suppress the body's hunger mechanisms.[4,5] These satiety-inducing effects are pronounced, lasting several hours after a meal. And when appetite isn't driven by hunger, food choices can more easily be made based on rationale rather than on impulse. This is why studies have consistently shown that when people are left to make their own nutritional decisions, those who consume higher amounts of protein take in significantly fewer calories than those who don't.

Lastly, protein is "insulin friendly." If you remember, insulin acts as a storage hormone. While its primary purpose is to neutralize blood sugar, insulin also is responsible for shuttling fat into fat cells. As insulin levels rise, so does the potential for fat deposition. Protein, however, has only a modest impact on insulin secretion. In fact, certain amino acids in protein stimulate the release of glucagon, a hormone that opposes insulin and keeps it in check. The end result: Your body is more apt to burn fat than to store it.

HOW MUCH PROTEIN DO YOU NEED?

So now we come to the million dollar question: "How much protein do you need in your diet?" It's an issue that's caused a great deal of controversy in nutrition circles. According to the United States Department of Agriculture, protein requirements are quite modest. Based on their Recommended Dietary Allowance (RDA), intake should equate to a little less than 4/10 of a gram of protein per pound of body weight. Thus, a person weighing 150 pounds would consume about 60 grams of protein a day—the equivalent of two skinless chicken breasts.

The RDA, however, has a major flaw in its design: it bases protein requirements on the average couch potato. While this is fine if you want to be an average couch potato, it has little relevance if your goal is to look great naked. In truth, those who aspire to optimize body composition do indeed require more protein than what is prescribed in the RDA.[6] Significantly more!

For physically active individuals (specifically those involved in exercise programs), studies have consistently shown optimal intake to be about 8/10 of a gram of protein per pound of body weight (roughly double the RDA).[7,8] The reasons are twofold: First, during exercise, amino acids are oxidized for fuel at an accelerated rate.[9] Depending on the intensity and duration of training, these amino acids can supply up to 10 percent of the body's energy needs. What's more, the stresses associated with physical activity cause an increased breakdown of body proteins, leaving the body in a catabolic state. The only way to reverse these effects and promote an anabolic environment is by consuming additional dietary protein, over and above RDA guidelines.[10,11] Abide by the RDA and you'll be breaking down body proteins at a faster rate than they can be replenished.

The benefits of a protein-rich diet also extend to the sedentary population. As previously discussed, protein has specific metabolic properties. By promoting satiety and inducing thermogenesis, it causes you to eat less and burn more. Over time, the caloric deficit created by these factors really adds up, helping to keep you leaner than with a "traditional" diet.

A higher protein intake is especially important when you're trying to lose weight.[12] During stringent dieting, there is a tendency for your body to break down protein stores into glucose (through a process called gluconeogenesis) so that the brain and other tissues have adequate fuel.[13] Since skeletal muscle is not necessary for sustenance (as opposed to the internal organs and other protein-based tissues), it is the primary bodily tissue to be cannibalized. The only way to counteract this occurrence is by consuming extra protein. Keeping protein intake high helps to preserve lean tissue, preventing the negative consequences of muscle wasting.[14]

Taking all factors into account, daily protein intake should correspond to approximately one gram of protein per pound of body weight. This provides a margin of safety, ensuring you will continue to build proteins at a faster rate than you break them down. There really is no downside to the approach: Taking in a little extra protein won't hurt; not getting enough surely will. As a frame of reference, 4 ounces of lean meat, chicken, or fish (about the size of your fist) contains roughly 30 grams of protein.

When calculating protein intake, figures should be based on "ideal" body weight rather than on actual body weight (if you are at maintenance, these numbers will be the same). Your ideal body weight has nothing to do with any medical charts or body mass index. No one, be it your doctor, nutritionist, or significant other, can tell you what you should weigh. Ideal body weight is purely a function of how *you* want to look. For example, if you want to weigh 150 pounds, protein intake should equate to approximately 150 grams per day. If a weight of 200 pounds is desired, consume 200 grams. Whatever number you choose, just make sure it is realistic for your body type.

On a cautionary note, you must guard against the temptation for overindulgence. It is not uncommon to see people ingest enormous quantities of protein in the thought that, "If a little is good, more must be better." Bodybuilders often subscribe to this misguided philosophy and gorge themselves with protein-based foods and supplements (one popular bodybuilder claims to ingest as much as 1,000 grams of protein a day!). Unfortunately, the body only has a limited capacity to utilize protein and there's no way to store it for future use. Beyond a certain threshold, hormones such as glucagon and catecholamines exert a counterregulatory effect, inhibiting any further protein synthesis.[15] Once this saturation point is reached, additional protein is of no use to the body and undergoes the same fate as carbohydrate: It is either burned as energy or converted into glycogen or fat.

Further, many popular fad diets (such as the 40-30-30 plan, among others) make the mistake of calculating protein intake as a percentage of total calories. The problem with this approach is that it fails to account for individual variances in protein requirements. If a fixed percent is used, there's a tendency to underestimate protein during periods of caloric restriction (i.e., weight loss) and overestimate protein con-

The High-Protein Myth

One of the biggest nutritional fallacies is that a diet high in protein places undue stress on the kidneys. This has long been a battle cry of the "anti-carb diet" crowd. Some in the medical establishment have even gone so far as to warn that if protein consumption exceeds baseline levels, you'll readily develop renal dysfunction and end up on dialysis. These scare tactics have raised concern over any diet that deviates from RDA guidelines.

The supposed association between protein intake and renal dysfunction is related to the intricacies of protein metabolism. During digestion, a complex sequence of events takes place where amino acids are *deaminated* (i.e., the amino group is removed). A by-product of this occurrence is the production and release of ammonia—a toxic substance—in the body. Luckily, ammonia doesn't remain in the body for long. The majority of it is rapidly converted into the relatively nontoxic, highly soluble substance urea, which is transported to the kidneys for excretion.[16]

In theory, a large buildup of urea can overtax the kidneys, impairing their ability to carry out vital functions. It has been well documented that a diet high in protein exacerbates kidney failure in those on dialysis; in contrast, protein restriction tends to alleviate the condition.[17] Given these findings, higher protein diets are generally contraindicated for anyone with existing kidney problems.

On the other hand, assuming you have normal renal function, there is no evidence that a diet high in protein is detrimental to the kidneys. Rather, published data shows that healthy kidneys are readily able to filter out urea; any excess is simply excreted in the urine.[18] Any alterations in renal size and function are merely normal physiological adaptations that aren't associated with any adverse effects.[19,20,21]

These results also have been confirmed empirically. Consider that, over the past century, millions of athletes have consumed large quantities of protein (as much as ten times the recommended daily allowance!) without ill effect. They'll scoff down chicken breasts by the dozen and drink protein shakes galore. Surely, if high-protein diets caused kidney disease, all of these athletes would be on dialysis by now. Yet, by all accounts, no reported renal abnormalities have been directly attributable to an increased intake of protein.[22]

sumption in cases of caloric surplus (i.e., bulking up). The bottom line is that protein percentages are, for all intents and purposes, of no consequence; intake should be based solely on ideal body weight.

FOOD COMBINING HYPE

Some nutritionists have postulated that protein and carbs should never be consumed at the same meal—a theory called food combining. The standard food combining protocol consists of fruit in the morning, fruit and a salad for lunch, vegetables and either a starch or protein food for dinner, and fruit again for a late-night snack. Suffice it to say, popular combinations such as eggs and toast, meat and potatoes, and fish and pasta are explicitly off-limits.

Although the genesis of food combining can be traced back to the nineteenth century, its most prominent modern-day promoter was Dr. Herbert Shelton. In recent years, Harvey Diamond, Suzanne Somers, and Marilu Henner have each popularized Shelton's views in bestselling books, bringing food combining into the mainstream.

The central premise behind food combining is based on the fact that the digestion of protein and carbs require different pH levels: Protein thrives in an acidic environment while carbs require a more alkaline milieu. According to food combining proponents, eating these foods at the same time neutralizes stomach acids and therefore prevents proper nutrient assimilation. Without a means to be metabolized, the nutrients simply putrefy and rot in the stomach. Over time, there is a buildup of toxic waste material (called toxemia), which ultimately causes the body to store excess fat.

The truth is, however, the food combining theory has no scientific basis. There isn't a shred of evidence that any negative complications are directly attributable to eating protein and carbs in the same meal. In fact, it has repeatedly been shown in clinically controlled studies that mixed diets are an excellent means to improve health and sustain weight loss.[23]

The concept of toxemia is, in itself, flawed. Nutrients can't rot in the stomach. Once ingested, they are either assimilated or eliminated. Whatever your body can't digest passes through to the colon and is excreted in the feces. Except for constipation, there simply is no mechanism by which food can remain in your system in a semi-degraded form for an extended period of time (if constipation is a problem, the likely cause is a lack of dietary fiber, not food combining).

Along the same lines, toxic waste cannot turn into fat—it's a physiologic impossibility. In order for foods to be stored in adipose tissue (i.e., fat cells), they must first be broken down and then converted into triglycerides. If a food is left undigested, it can't be absorbed–period. And if a food can't be absorbed, then it can't be metabolized into a triglyceride (or anything else, for that matter).

Epidemiologic evidence would tell you there is no reason to separate your intake of nutrients. Throughout history, humans have eaten an endless variety of foods without ill effect. The Japanese, whose meals are based on combining protein and carbs, have among the lowest rates of obesity in the world (at least they did until fast food began invading their culture!).

Still not convinced? Well, consider the typical bodybuilding diet. In their precompetition phase, bodybuilders often subsist on nothing but chicken and rice (eaten at the same sitting). According to food combining proponents, these athletes should all be fat from their regimens. Instead, the opposite happens; they manage to attain body fat percentages as low as 4 percent!

There are practical reasons why it's actually beneficial to consume protein and carbs together. For one, protein synthesis is mediated by insulin and the primary nutrient responsible for insulin secretion is . . . you guessed it, carbohydrate! By eating protein with carbohydrate, the body has a steady source of amino acids along with the necessary insulin to facilitate their uptake into cells. In fact, anabolism has been shown to be about 20 percent greater when protein is consumed with each meal in contrast to one or two daily feedings.[24]

And food combining is energetically wasteful. When you eat only a couple of large protein-based meals a day, there is a tendency for the body to utilize protein for energy, rather than for tissue-building purposes. Since it's inefficient and costly to use protein as a fuel source, this strategy makes little sense.

WHAT ABOUT QUALITY?

Much has been made about the qualitative aspects of various proteins. Muscle magazines routinely publish articles on the subject, using terms such as biological value (BV), protein efficiency ratio (PER), and protein digestibility corrected amino acid score (PDCAAS) to tout the benefits of one type of protein over another. For the majority of people, however, all of this talk about protein quality is much ado about nothing.

The quality of a protein is largely a function of its composition of essential amino acids, both in terms of quantity and proportion. A "complete" protein contains a full complement of essential amino acids in the approximate amounts needed by the body. Conversely, proteins that are low in one or more of the essential amino acids are considered "incomplete."

With the exception of gelatin, all animal-based proteins (meats, dairy products, eggs, etc.) are complete proteins. So assuming you eat a variety of animal-based foods (and follow my protocol for consuming one gram of protein per pound of body weight), qualitative issues are moot; you are assured of getting all the essential amino acids you need for optimal development.

Vegetable-based proteins, on the other hand, lack various essential amino acids, which makes them incomplete. For lacto-ovo vegetarians, this isn't really an issue since protein can be obtained from eggs and dairy products, which have a full complement of amino acids. But vegans have to be a little more careful here. They need to eat food in the right combinations to ensure that adequate essential amino acids are procured through dietary means. For instance, grains are limited in lysine and threonine, while legumes are low in methionine. Combining the two offsets the weaknesses of each, thereby helping to prevent a deficiency.

THE BEST PROTEIN FOODS

There is a prevailing misconception that a diet high in protein results in an inordinate intake of unhealthy saturated fat. The popularity of low-carb diets has only served to fuel this fire. Ketogenic gurus tout high-fat foods such as bacon, T-bone steaks, hard cheeses, and whole milk as viable dietary options and even encourage their consumption. Consequently, protein-rich foods have become synonymous with the intake of artery-clogging fats.

The truth is, however, "higher protein" does not necessarily mean "higher fat." There is no reason that protein intake must be derived from fatty foods. In fact, many quality protein sources contain little, if any, saturated fat. By simply choosing the right foods, a higher protein diet can be maintained with minimal effect on fat consumption. And as you'll see, my approach is to encourage consumption of lean sources of protein. It's relatively easy to meet protein requirements with whole foods. For example, a 4-ounce chicken breast contains about 30 grams of protein; so does one cup of tofu; three large eggs; and a little over half a can of albacore tuna. By consuming any combination of these foods, you'll easily achieve the necessary protein intake to maintain a positive balance.

So what are the best lean protein sources? Well, many terrific options exist—enough to satisfy almost everyone's taste buds. Let's discuss the myriad options.

Poultry

Poultry is a protein staple. It has long been a favorite of bodybuilders and other physique-oriented athletes. Turkey and chicken, in particular, provide excellent protein quality with low levels of saturated fat. Duck and goose, while not quite as lean, still make good choices. Other types of fowl such as pheasant and quail have a slightly "gamey" taste, providing a low-fat way to add variety to your diet.

There is one caveat to poultry consumption: only eat the white meat. The dark meat (found primarily in the drumsticks and wings) is actually extremely fatty, containing about as much saturated fat as chuck steak. So when shopping for poultry, make sure the meat comes from the breast. This is especially important when buying ground poultry; eating a turkey burger made from dark meat is no healthier than eating a regular hamburger!

The way you cook poultry also is an issue. If the meat has skin, make sure you remove it *before* you begin cooking (a 3.5-ounce serving of turkey skin has 39 grams of fat—most of it saturated!). Heat causes the underlying fat from the skin to seep into the meat. You're left with a meal that has significantly more saturated fat than a comparably prepared skinless breast.

Seafood

Seafood is another great protein source. Many types of fish (such as flounder, cod, and grouper) are virtually devoid of fat. Others (especially the cold-water variety such as salmon, mackerel, and trout) contain ample amounts of healthy unsaturated fats that are essential to well-being (the benefits of which will be discussed in Chapter 6). And shellfish such as shrimp, scallops, and lobster are low in fat and delicious.

One of the best things about seafood is that it provides a tremendous amount of dietary diversity. Each fish has its own unique taste and can be prepared in a multitude of ways. Unlike other meats, you can eat seafood almost every day and never get bored. With so many different species, the possibilities are virtually endless.

Fish can also be eaten raw. Sushi and sashimi, long a favorite in the Far East, are becoming increasingly popular in Western society. With their combination of exotic flavors and chic presentation, these delights can be enjoyed on a regular basis. Make sure you get sushi or sashimi from a reputable place, though. Poor-quality sushi or sashimi can contain parasites such as tapeworm. If eaten, these parasites invade your internal organs, causing a host of unpleasant gastrointestinal problems.

Be especially careful when eating shellfish such as clams and oysters. These mollusks are bottom-feeders and therefore tend to carry a high concentration of infectious agents and toxins. Thus, if consumed raw or undercooked, there is a heightened risk of diseases such as typhoid fever, salmonellosis, shigellosis, campylobacteriosis, cholera, Norwalk-like gastroenteritis, and hepatitis A.[25] The best advice is to limit these foods to occasional consumption, and preferably eat them only when fully cooked.

Beef

Beef has benefits over and above its protein value. Namely, it is rich in creatine, an amino acid compound that's integrally involved in anaerobic exercise (like weight training). Although the body can manufacture creatine, many people don't produce enough to fill their creatine stores—as much as 80 percent of the population, by some accounts.[26] If you fall into this category, consuming creatine through food sources enhances its storage in cells, improving both the quality of your workout and physique.[27]

And despite its reputation for being unhealthy, beef actually can be a relatively lean source of protein—provided you choose the right types of meat. Certainly, porterhouse and chuck are very fatty cuts; anything on the bone or with a lot of marbling will fall into this category. But several cuts are actually quite lean: sirloin, flank, and round steaks contain only moderate amounts of fat.

Game meats such as buffalo or venison are even better alternatives. Due to their increased activity levels and free-range diet, they tend to carry very low levels of adipose and increased amounts of healthy essential fats.

When buying red meat, look for organically raised livestock. These animals have been allowed to graze in the wild rather than being fattened up on commercial grains. What you get is a leaner cut of meat that contains a healthier profile of essential fats. You'll pay a little more, but it's worth it.

No matter what type of beef you choose, make sure to trim all visible fat before cooking. This will ensure that as little as possible seeps into the meat. If you buy lean cuts, most of the fat will be around the edges, so it should be relatively easy to cut most of it out.

Beans

Generally, vegetables contain only small amounts of protein. The notable exception is beans. Although they tend to be somewhat low in methionine, beans contain a fairly good mix of essential amino acids. Moreover, there are many different types from which to choose (including black beans, lima beans, kidney beans, and others), providing a great deal of possibilities for adding variety to your diet.

Of all the various kinds of beans, soy deserves special mention. Due to its purported health-promoting effects, soy consumption has gone through the roof. There is now a plethora of soy-containing products on the market, including soy milk, soy energy bars, soy meats, and even soy ice cream. And if that's not enough, you can buy soy in powders or in pill form and get a quick fix of soy, anytime, anywhere.

And, as opposed to so many nutritional products, soy isn't just a lot of hype. Studies have shown that regular soy consumption helps to lower the bad LDL cholesterol and raise the good HDL cholesterol.[28] This is attributed to its content of phytoestrogens—naturally occurring plant compounds that have weak estrogenic properties. Since cholesterol is a primary factor in cardiovascular disease, soy unquestionably has heart-healthy benefits. On the flip side of the coin, however, there

The Ongoing Study of Soy

There is some evidence that soy can alleviate many of the symptoms associated with menopause.[29,30,31] Due to its phytoestrogens, soy has been shown to reduce the incidence of hot flashes and night sweats. And by suppressing the activity of osteoclasts (whose job is to break down bone tissue), these same phytoestrogens can even help to mitigate bone loss.[32] Since there is a profound increase in bone resorption during menopause—as much as 3 percent per year—soy can be of significant benefit for the mature woman.

Less clear is the claim that soy is an anticarcinogen. On one hand, several studies do show that soy helps to reduce the risk of various forms of cancer.[33] Other studies, however, suggest that soy might actually promote tumor growth.[34] Because of the phytoestrogens, breast tumors have actually increased in size when soy was given to women with existing breast cancer. It's difficult to know what to make of these conflicting reports, but the fact that there's even the potential for increasing cancer risk is cause for alarm.

There also is some concern that a high intake of soy might suppress immune function. Some studies have shown that genistein, one of the soy isoflavones, has an adverse effect on the thymus gland.[35] The thymus is responsible for the production of T cells, one of the primary compounds involved in initiating an immune response, and any reduction in T cells can impair your body's ability to fight off disease.

are questions about the safety of soy for various populations, including those with suppressed immune function and those with preexisting history of cancer, particularly in the breast.

Given the contradictory research regarding soy's effect on many areas of health, it is prudent to take a moderate approach to soy intake: Include soy as part of your diet but refrain from consuming it on a daily basis. Three or four ounces of soy products several days a week should be considered an upper limit, especially if there is a history of breast cancer. Until further studies clarify the facts, it's best to err on the side of caution. While soy's therapeutic properties show a great deal of promise, there are still more questions that need to be answered before it can be labeled as a nutritional cure-all.

Finally, beans are notorious for causing flatulence. This is due to their content of *oligosaccharides.* In order to be digested, oligosaccharides require the enzyme alpha-galactosidase. Humans, however, don't possess this enzyme. So once ingested, oligosaccharides enter the colon intact and the end result is excess bowel gas.[36]

If this is a problem for you, consider taking a supplement such as Beano. These products supply the alpha-galactosidase enzyme, facilitating better digestion of legumes. They are available in convenient tablets and easy-to-use drops, and are generally well tolerated by most people.

Dairy

Dairy products such as milk, cheese, and yogurt are viable options for satisfying your protein requirements. They have balanced amino acids profiles and are high in the minerals potassium and magnesium. They also are rich in calcium and vitamin D, thereby helping to promote strong bones and teeth.

However, dairy products contain higher amounts of sugars than other protein sources—the main sugar being lactose. Lactose is a disaccharide, composed of glucose and galactose. Unfortunately, about 25 percent of the population lack the enzyme responsible for breaking down lactose and therefore are unable to properly digest dairy. This condition, called lactose intolerance, can cause abdominal bloating, diarrhea, and stomach cramps. Certain ethnic groups including Asians and African-Americans have much higher rates of lactose intolerance—more than 80 percent, by some estimates. What's more, many others are "quasi" lactose intolerant, having the ability to tolerate only small quantities of dairy.

But even if you are lactose intolerant, dairy still can be included as part of your diet. Tolerance to lactose can often be improved by starting out with small amounts and gradually increasing consumption over time. Under normal circumstances, your body will increase its enzyme production, allowing you to eventually tolerate dairy products without a problem.

You also can opt for one of the many lactose-free dairy products now on the market. Alternatively, consider taking caplets such as Lactaid or Dairy Ease. They can be chewed or swallowed before you eat a lactose-rich dish and improve your body's capacity for its digestion.

It is also important to note that dairy products tend to be high in saturated fats. Thus, it's best to choose low-fat dairy alternatives. Stick to products that contain 2 percent fat or less.

Eggs

Eggs might be the best protein source of all. Due to a favorable profile of essential amino acids, eggs have the highest biological value (a popular measure of protein quality) of any protein source. Their score is so nearly perfect, in fact, that egg protein is often the standard by which all other proteins are judged.

From a protein perspective, the whites of eggs are as perfect a food as there is. They contain 4 grams of protein per large white with no saturated fat—nothing but pure protein. Egg whites make terrific omelets and can be used in many recipes to enhance the protein content (and taste!) of other foods.

Egg yolks, although protein rich (one yolk contains about 4 grams of protein), provide somewhat of a nutritional conundrum. On one hand, they are a good source of various healthy nutrients including lecithin and essential fatty acids. On the other hand, they contain a fair amount of unhealthy saturated fats (approximately 2 grams per large egg) that negatively affect body composition.

Given these facts, the consumption of egg yolks should be based on your nutritional goals. If you want to lose weight, limit intake to one yolk per day. Adding a yolk to several egg whites can give an omelet flavor without having much impact on the total amount of calories and saturated fat in your diet as a whole. Alternatively, if your goal is to bulk up, you can take a more liberal stance. In this case, several yolks a day can help to supply valuable nutrients to fuel growth.

As with meats, it's best to buy organic eggs—especially if you want to eat the yolks. Chickens that roam free and eat as they choose produce eggs with higher levels of lecithin and essential fatty acids than those produced in commercial egg farms.

If you just want the whites, several companies sell them in cartons that resemble milk containers. These are real whites that undergo pasteurization to preserve freshness. They are extremely convenient (taking away the hassle of separating out the yolk) and taste great. I highly recommend them.

ARE PROTEIN POWDERS BENEFICIAL?

If, for any reason, you have trouble getting enough protein from whole foods, you might consider using a protein powder. Understand that you don't *need* protein powders to have a great physique. In most instances, protein needs can easily be satisfied by consuming whole foods. But protein powders do provide good utility, conveniently allowing you to get a protein-based meal in a matter of minutes.

There are a wide variety of powders on the market, derived from just about every available protein source. The two I generally recommend are whey and casein, preferably a blend of the two. These milk-based proteins each provide unique benefits and, because they digest at different speeds, are complementary when consumed in conjunction with each other. Most of the lactose is removed so they shouldn't pose much of a problem for the lactose intolerant. Just add them to water, juice, or whole foods for a power-packed meal.

It should be noted that protein powders aren't magic formulas for building muscle. Contrary to claims made by various supplement manufacturers, you can't simply suck down a protein drink, sit back, and watch your muscles grow. While this might make good ad copy, it simply doesn't translate into reality. Adding quality muscle mass requires a combination of adequate calories, dietary protein (in accordance with your body weight), and intense weight training. To the extent that you get these factors right, your muscles will develop to their ultimate potential.

Summary of the Look Great Naked Diet Protein Protocol

1. Consume approximately 1 gram of protein per pound of ideal body weight daily.
2. Whenever possible, consume protein with carbs.
3. Eat a variety of lean protein sources. If you're a vegan, consume combinations of legumes and grains, preferably in the same meal.
4. Consume soy in moderation.
5. If you have difficulty getting enough protein from whole foods, consider taking a high-quality protein powder.

CHAPTER 6

The Skinny on Fat

Fat is a necessary part of your daily diet—just as important, in its own way, as carbohydrates and protein. As with these other nutrients, the question is not whether you *should* consume fat, but rather *what kinds* and *how much* you need to consume. In this chapter, you'll find guidelines for fat consumption that are surprisingly easy to follow (in fact, there are just six simple steps, summarized at the end of the chapter). Once you adopt my guidelines, you'll find yourself *automatically* making food choices to avoid "bad" fats and to get the "good" fats. Developing these new habits is essential for optimizing body composition.

As many people are now aware, excessive saturated fat in the diet inevitably will lead to an increase of fatty tissue in the body. In large part, this is because the concentration of calories is so high. There are nine calories in each gram of fat—about double the number of calories found in a single gram of carbohydrates or protein. All other factors aside, this tells you right away that you have to expend twice the amount of energy to "work off" the calories you get from fat.

But there are many other factors to be considered. Fat has its pluses as well as its minuses. For instance, fat helps to keep your hunger in check—a vital factor in dietary adherence. Fat also contributes to cellular health, affecting not only interior tissues but also the appearance of your skin, hair, and nails.

When you consume excessive dietary fat, however, you run the risk of many adverse effects. Some fats, as you'll see, have a "hardening" effect on cell membranes, which inhibits cellular function. Overconsumption of "bad fats" can also raise the set point of your body, which makes it more difficult for you to maintain optimum weight and lean body mass. Also, some of the "bad fats" actually have a life-threatening effect—dangerously elevating your risk of heart disease and quite possibly increasing your risk of certain kinds of cancer as well.

What I recommend in the LGN Diet is, first, that you carefully measure your intake of dietary fat. I'll give you some simple formulas for calculating how much you should be getting on a daily basis. Second, I'll help you understand the differences between different kinds of fat at the molecular level and how these differences affect your weight and health. (Molecular structure actually affects the way those fats are incorporated in your body and utilized by your cells.) Third, I'll list the best sources of dietary fat, making it easy to determine the "good" from the "bad." By the time you've finished reading this chapter, you'll have all the ammunition you need to steer away from fats that lead to weight gain and increased health risks and to choose food sources that help you improve cellular health, guard against heart disease, and keep your energy at optimal levels.

THE FAT-FREE PARADOX

For many years, the medical establishment cautioned that dietary fat was the enemy, a surefire ticket to a life of corpulence and ill health. "Eat fat and you'll get fat," they cried, and a legion of health-conscious consumers listened. "Fat-free" became a buzzword destined to sell products: Stores couldn't get fat-free foods onto their shelves fast enough; fat-free cookbooks rapidly made their way to the bestseller charts; and wellness spas thrived by trumpeting their fat-free menus. It all seemed to be going so well . . .

But a funny thing happened. Despite cutting back significantly on fat consumption, Americans keep getting fatter and fatter! The number of people considered overweight has ballooned (no pun intended) to about two-thirds of the population, with more than 20 percent deemed clinically obese. Clearly, it isn't just fat intake accounting for our ever-expanding waistlines. To appreciate why, it's necessary to unlock some of the mysteries of how dietary fat is processed by the body.

Fats, also known as lipids, are classified into two basic categories: saturated and unsaturated. While there are many subtypes within these categories, all fats have one thing in common: They are made up of chains of carbon and hydrogen atoms. The chains range between four and twenty-four carbon atoms with the hydrogens surrounding the carbons. Chains of four to six carbons are called short-chain fatty acids, chains of eight to twelve carbons are called medium-chain fatty acids, and those above twelve carbons are called long-chain fatty acids. By far, it's the long-chain fatty acids that predominate in foods, accounting for more than 90 percent of fat intake in the average American diet.

The Dangers of Fat

Theoretically, it is beneficial to limit fat consumption. The primary reason is that fat is calorically dense; each gram contains nine calories. Do the math and you'll see that you have to eat more than twice the amount of protein or carbs (which both have only four calories per gram) to get the same number of calories from a given portion of fat. And since energy balance (calories in versus calories out) is the overriding determinant in weight management, watching your fat intake is a sound nutritional strategy.

The Benefits of Fat

Extremely low-fat diets are counterproductive. If nothing else, fats are an essential nutrient and play a vital role in many bodily functions. They are involved in cushioning your internal organs for protection, aiding in the absorption of vitamins, and facilitating the production of cell membranes, hormones, and prostaglandins. Physiologically, it would be impossible to survive without the inclusion of fats in your diet.

Fats are important on other levels, too. For one, they improve the palatability of food, a fact that generally leads to better dietary adherence.[1] After all, who's going to stick with a diet if the food tastes bad? While you don't necessarily have to eat like a gourmet, meals should at least be enjoyable, something you look forward to (or at least don't abhor). The inclusion of dietary fat contributes to that enjoyment, making you more inclined to remain dedicated to your nutritional regimen.

Fats also play a role in satiety, exerting their influence in two distinct ways. First, when fats reach the stomach, they stimulate a hormone called enterogastrone, which inhibits the passage of food through the gastrointestinal system. Thus, food stays in the gut longer, slowing digestion. What's more, the hormone CCK is released. If you remember, one of the roles of CCK is to signal the brain that your stomach is full, keeping hunger in check. In combination, these events help to curb food cravings, reducing the urge to binge.

And the consumption of fats even plays a role in your outward appearance. Since your body's number-one priority is survival, it will use fats for essential functions before cosmetic issues. With a deficiency, dermatologic complications arise: your skin gets flaky; your nails become brittle and break off; and your hair dries out, losing its luster. Only by consuming adequate dietary fat can these conditions be reversed.

Rather than looking to cut out dietary fat, you should instead focus on the quality of the fats that you eat. There are good and bad fats, and consuming the right ones in the right amounts can have a profound effect on body composition.

THE BAD: SATURATED FATS

Saturated fats, abundant in many meats and dairy products, are unhealthy fats. As a rule, they serve no biological purpose and can cause a host of harmful effects in the body.

Structure

The detriments of saturated fats can be traced back to their structure (stay with me on this as it will all make sense shortly). As previously discussed, all fats are composed of a linked chain of carbon atoms surrounded by hydrogen atoms. With saturated fats, there is a hydrogen atom on both sides of every carbon. In effect, the carbons are "saturated" with hydrogens. The result is a molecule that resembles a straight caterpillar, which allows the fats to pack together tightly and thereby remain solid at room temperature.

This "straight caterpillar" conformation is detrimental to body composition. You see, your body is programmed to interact with molecules that have certain shapes and, unfortunately, a straight caterpillar isn't one of them. These fats therefore have no utility; if not utilized immediately for energy, they're shuttled into fat cells for long-term storage. This has been demonstrated in research studies: Given the same caloric intake, eating saturated fats results in a greater body-fat deposition than either protein or carbs.[2,3]

LDL: The "Bad Cholesterol"

Saturated fats also elevate cholesterol levels.[4] Under normal circumstances, cholesterol isn't the culprit that it's often made out to be. In fact, it takes part in a host of biological functions: It is a constituent in cell membranes, acts as a precursor to many hormones (including the sex hormones estrogen and testosterone), and forms the basis of bile salts that aid in the digestion and absorption of fat and fat-soluble vitamins in the intestine. However, when cholesterol levels become elevated, major problems arise. Research shows that high blood cholesterol is a direct precursor to heart attacks and strokes.[5] The consensus among most medical professionals is that it's a primary factor in cardiac risk.

Cholesterol is a waxy, fatlike substance that is taken up through protein-based compounds called *lipoproteins* for use in various target tissues. In effect, lipoproteins act as little shuttle buses that carry cholesterol to and from cells. While there are several different classifications of lipoproteins, the most notable are the low-density lipoproteins (LDL) and high-density lipoproteins (HDL).

LDL, the "bad cholesterol," is the one commonly associated with cardiovascular disease. When excessive amounts of LDL circulate in the bloodstream, they attach themselves to the lining of the arteries. Over time, these cholesterol deposits become oxidized (think of rust on the inside of a pipe), causing localized inflammation and arterial plaque. Plaque buildup can get so large that it clogs the artery, impeding blood flow. In severe cases, the artery can become completely blocked, cutting off circulation to the heart, brain, legs, or other organs.

Saturated fat intake directly increases blood levels of the "bad" LDL cholesterol by decreasing production of LDL receptors in the liver.[6,7] These receptors are the gateways that allow cholesterol to be cleared from your circulatory system. Without a port of entry, cholesterol can't enter into liver cells for removal so it just keeps circulating in the bloodstream (think of little LDL shuttle buses that have no destination). Eventually, the cholesterol attaches to the walls of your arteries, initiating the inflammatory process that leads to fatty plaque formation.

As a point of interest, it should be noted that cholesterol-laden foods have little if any effect on blood cholesterol. This is due to the body's ability to increase and decrease its own internal cholesterol production based on the amount of cholesterol consumed in the diet: Eat more cholesterol, your body produces less; eat less, your body produces more. (It should be noted that a small percentage of the population called "hyperresponders" have a defect in this feedback loop and, for these people, cholesterol intake must be kept to a minimum.)

On top of everything, saturated fats have even been implicated in certain types of cancers.[8] Some research suggests that they promote tumors of the breast, prostate, and bladder.[9,10,11] Although a direct link to these cancers has not been firmly established, there's reasonable cause to believe a connection exists. And a strong correlation has been found between saturated fat intake and colorectal cancer, with most evidence pointing to significant increases in risk.[12,13,14]

There are many subtypes of saturated fats, and some are more harmful than others. Unfortunately, most fatty foods contain a mixture of saturated fats, making it impossible to consume one without consuming the others. For example, stearic acid is considered relatively benign. It has almost no impact on cholesterol or other cardiovascular markers. Lauric, myristic, and palmitic acids, on the other hand, are renowned for their hypercholesteremic effects and have been associated with an increased risk of mortality. Bottom line: Learn to read labels and choose foods containing little or no saturated fat. Most products clearly list saturated fat content, so the amount isn't difficult to ascertain.

Saturated Fat and Your Set Point

Saturated fats have a tendency to collect in cell membranes, hardening them and thereby desensitizing the cell to external stimuli and inhibiting cellular processes. This is particularly damaging to muscles as it makes their cells less responsive to insulin.[15,16] And as previously stated, impaired insulin function leads to a host of negative consequences, not the least of which is increased fat deposition. There also is a negative effect on leptin, with decreases in both production and sensitivity.[17] As a result, prolonged consumption of foods high in saturated fats can also lead to a raised set point.

THE GOOD: UNSATURATED FATS

Unsaturated fats are healthier fats. As opposed to the saturated variety, these fats contain one or more *double bonds* (double strong bonds that link hydrogen to the carbons) in their carbon chain. For each double bond, there is a loss of two hydrogen atoms from the chain. The end result is a fat that's no longer saturated with hydrogens (hence the moniker "unsaturated"). Because of their structure, which allows the carbon chain to kink, these fats cannot aggregate and therefore remain liquid at room temperature.

Monounsaturated Fats

Fats with one double bond are called monounsaturated fats (MUFAs), the predominant one being oleate, an omega-9 fatty acid. Olive oil is the most abundant source of MUFAs, with more than 75 percent of its calories coming from oleate. Other foods high in monounsaturates include almonds, avocados, pecans, and pistachio nuts.

Until recently, MUFAs were thought to be "neutral" fats because they didn't appear to have an effect—either positive or negative—on blood cholesterol levels. As it turns out, however, olive oil is actually a functional food, possessing many therapeutic qualities.[18] It contains an array of healthy compounds (including phytosterols, polyphenols, and sqaulene) that act as potent antioxidants, which serve to prevent disease states and improve body composition.[19] (See Chapter 13 for a detailed discussion of antioxidants.)

The benefits of MUFAs have been clearly demonstrated in studies of the Mediterranean diet. In these diets, consumption of fats is around 40 percent of total calories, with the majority of fat calories coming from olive oil.[20] With such a high fat intake, standard nutritional theory would predict a high rate of cardiovascular disease. But this isn't the case. In fact, the Greeks, Italians, and other southern Europeans actually have reduced rates of heart attacks and strokes! In looking to explain this paradox, scientists determined that the healthful effects of the Mediterranean diet were largely due to its high composition of olive oil.[21]

Monounsaturates have additional benefits on body tissues. Namely, they help to maintain fluidity in cell membranes, allowing hormones and other chemical messengers to readily penetrate the cells. This has wide-ranging effects, from increasing muscle protein synthesis to improving insulin sensitivity to enhancing fat burning.[22]

All things considered, monounsaturates should be readily consumed in your diet. Replacing fats from saturated sources with those from monounsaturated sources is an excellent strategy to improve body composition and health without compromising taste.

Polyunsaturated Fats: Essential Fatty Acids

Fats with two or more double bonds are called polyunsaturated fats (PUFAs). There are two primary classes of PUFAs: omega-6 linoleate and omega-3 alpha-linoleate. Due to an absence of certain enzymes in the human body, we cannot manufacture these fats in our bodies and therefore PUFAs are an essential component in food. A PUFA deficiency ultimately causes a breakdown in cellular function, leading to a host of anomalies including bloody urine, fatty liver, and even reproductive disorders.

In addition to their cellular interactions, PUFAs have other physiologic benefits. Like the monounsaturates, they are integral components of cell membranes. Because of their multiple double-bond structure, PUFAs are the most fluid of all fats. When incorporated into membranes, they enhance permeability, helping to maintain optimal cell signaling.

It's important to realize, though, that omega-6 and omega-3 fatty acids aren't interchangeable. They have separate and distinct effects on bodily processes, many of them antagonistic of one another. And, for the most part, it's the omega-3s that are the most nutritionally beneficial.

OMEGA-3 ESSENTIAL FATTY ACIDS

Omega-3s exert a significant cardioprotective effect.[23] Not only do they inhibit the production of LDL (the "bad" form of cholesterol), but they also increase the output of HDL (the "good" cholesterol).[24,25] HDL acts as a cholesterol scavenger, carrying surplus cholesterol from the tissues back to the liver. Once it reaches the liver, cholesterol is either excreted in the feces or converted into bile acids, which are important compounds that act as emulsifying agents in the gut in the digestion of fats and oils. Plasma HDL concentrations are inversely related to coronary artery disease—the greater the amount of HDL, the lower the incidence of heart attacks and vice versa. This explains why replacing saturated fats with omega-3s on a calorie-for-calorie basis has been shown to reduce the risk of cardiovascular mortality by as much as 70 percent![26]

Perhaps the most underappreciated aspect of omega-3s is their impact on reducing body fat. That's right, eating the right fats can actually help to make you thin! Because of their utility on cells, the body prefers to use omega-3s to fuel cellular functions and won't store them as fat until these functions are satisfied.[27]

Omega-3s also have indirect influences on expediting fat loss. They act as fuel partitioners, directing fatty acids away from storage and toward oxidation. One of the ways this is accomplished is through enzyme regulation. Specifically, omega-3s help to increase the activity of fat-burning enzymes and suppress the activity of fat-storing enzymes.[28] The net effect is better fat metabolism and therefore improved body composition.

Additionally, omega-3s increase levels of a class of fat-burning compounds called uncoupling proteins (UCPs).[29] UCPs act on various bodily tissues to heighten thermogenesis, allowing calories to be burned off immediately as heat rather than stored as fat. Unfortunately, these substances are often suppressed, especially in those who are overweight.[30] By revving up UCP activity, PUFAs shift your body into a fat-burning mode, promoting a leaner physique.

OMEGA-3S AND YOUR SET POINT

Omega-3s even have a positive impact on leptin. They counteract the effects of saturated fats, increasing both leptin production and sensitivity.[31] This directly aids in long-term weight management, helping to keep your set point low.

Keeping a Balance: Omega-3s and Omega-6s

Omega-6s are precursors to an important group of compounds called eicosanoids, which are substances that have hormonelike actions in virtually every tissue in the body. Eicosanoids are classified into three different "series" that each has a specific purpose, with those in one series having opposing actions on those in another series. For instance, series 1 eicosanoids decrease inflammation, dilate blood vessels, and reduce blood clotting, while series 2 eicosanoids increase inflammation, constrict blood vessels, and promote blood clotting.

Given this yin/yang relationship, a delicate balance needs to be maintained between eicosanoids; an excess of one series over another becomes problematic. The overproduction of series 2 eicosanoids, in particular, is linked to many disease states, including hypertension, allergies, rheumatoid arthritis, stroke, and heart attack. Unfortunately, the human body has no reliable mechanism for maintaining this balance on its own.

Equilibrium in eicosanoid levels is primarily achieved through dietary means. Through a complex enzymatic reaction, omega-6 fatty acids obtained through food contribute to the formation of eicosanoids, particularly the series 2 variety. Omega-3s, on the other hand, exert a powerful counterregulatory influence over the omega-6s and suppress the formation of series 2 eicosanoids, keeping them in check. Based on eicosanoid theory, it's easy to see that a higher intake of omega-6 than omega-3 can have dire consequences. Sadly, the current Western diet has an omega-6 to omega-3 ratio that hovers in the range of about 20:1!

While research isn't yet definitive, scientists postulate that the appropriate omega-6 to omega-3 ratio is in the range of 4:1 or lower. Studies have shown that this ratio maintains equilibrium of the various eicosanoids, fine-tuning their ability to maintain optimal health. However, eicosanoids aren't the only issue here. Remember that omega-3s act as fuel partitioners, allowing fat to be burned rather than stored. They are the most biologically active of all fats and, therefore, provide the greatest metabolic benefits.

Taking everything into account, a ratio of 1:1 is generally a better bet. Realize that our Paleolithic ancestors, on whom our genetic pool is based, maintained a fairly equal balance of omega-6s to omega-3s.[32,33] Their diet consisted almost exclusively of lean wild meats, fish, vegetables, and fruits, all of which had a high omega-3 content.

Recent studies on Inuit Eskimos support a high omega-3 intake. The Inuits have one of the lowest incidences of heart attacks (one entire town didn't have a single case of cardiovascular disease throughout the 1970s!), yet they consume a very high percentage of their total calories from fat.[34] But guess where the fat calories come from? You got it, omega-3s. They survive on a diet of whale and seal blubber that supplies an average of 14 grams of omega-3s per day.[35] Bottom line is that there doesn't seem to be any downside to a ratio that favors omega-3s and the benefits are significant.

You *must* consume adequate amounts of the essential fats on a regular basis. Next to protein, they're the most important nutrients in your diet. Since omega-6s tend to be plentiful in foods, the focus should be on getting enough omega-3s to optimize body composition.

THE UGLY: TRANS FAT

There is one type of unsaturated fat called trans fat that should be avoided at all costs. Although technically unsaturated, trans fats actually behave very much like saturated fats. They are formed during a process in which vegetable oils are heated and exposed to hydrogen gas. This process, called *partial hydrogenation,* solidifies the oil, giving it certain desirable qualities—namely spreadability and increased shelf life. However, these benefits come at a price: hydrogenation destroys the healthy double carbon bonds of the oil, producing compounds that are foreign to the human body.

From a cardiovascular standpoint, trans fats can be considered the "anti-PUFAs." Their consumption has been shown to elevate blood levels of LDL (the "bad" cholesterol) and lower levels of HDL (the "good" cholesterol). This unhealthy combination makes trans fats even more detrimental than saturated fats (which at least don't decrease HDL).[36,37] It's no accident that the introduction of trans fats coincided with an epidemic of coronary heart disease in the Western world; researchers conclude that more than 30,000 premature deaths per year are attributable to their consumption.[38]

Trans fats also interfere with the *desaturation* of essential fats.[39] Since trans fats retain some of the characteristics of unsaturated fats (they are made from PUFAs), they bind to various enzymes. These enzymes mistakenly recognize the trans fat as a "healthy" PUFA, thereby blocking entry of omega-6 and omega-3 fatty acids into cells. This impairs your body's ability to use essential fats for cellular functions, leading to a host of negative complications.

Although all of their effects haven't been fully explained, it is speculated that trans fats might have carcinogenic properties. Since they are foreign to the human body, there is a greater likelihood of developing mutations—the precursors to the formation of cancers. Indeed, studies have shown evidence of an increased risk of colon cancer with trans fat intake—by some accounts greater than that of saturated fat.[40]

Trans fats have become increasingly popular in today's society, now making up approximately 8 percent of the average Western diet.[41] They are found in a wide array of processed foods. Margarine is perhaps the biggest culprit, with a whopping 60 percent of calories coming from trans fats. Salad dressings, doughnuts, potato chips, and cookies all tend to have high amounts, as do many fast-food items such as French fries and chicken nuggets. Apparently, manufacturers are more than willing to sacrifice nutritional value for convenience; you shouldn't be.

Recently, the Food and Drug Administration has ordered that trans fat content be included on food labels. However, at the time of this writing, compliance has been spotty, making it difficult to identify products that contain trans fats (this has led to their being nicknamed "phantom fats"). The best way to ensure you avoid them is to check ingredients. Stay away from anything with the words "partially hydrogenated," especially if it is one of the first items mentioned (ingredients are posted from highest concentration to lowest). Make the effort to cut these villains from your diet; it's one of the most important things you can do for your health and body.

DETERMINING OPTIMAL FAT INTAKE

Your total fat intake should be determined by adding the percentages from protein and carbohydrate in your diet together—whatever's left over is the percentage from fat. For example, if carbs equal 50 percent of calories and protein equals 30 percent of calories, then fat intake will be 20 percent. Since protein intake is a constant (based on ideal body weight), consumption of fat will be proportional to the amount of dietary carbs: If carbs are higher, fat will be lower and vice versa. It's simple mathematics.

While you only need several grams to fulfill bodily requirements and prevent a deficiency, most people tend to function best with at least 15 to 20 percent of calories from fat. And although no upper limit has been established, it seems that consuming more than 40 percent or so is unnecessary and perhaps counterproductive. As long as you stick to the recommendations provided, your intake will invariably fall within these limits.

Helpful Hint

You need to be very cognizant of your portions of fat-based foods—more so than with any other nutrient. Remember that fat is extremely energy dense, containing nine calories per gram. Therefore, small amounts add up to lots of calories, and miscalculating how much you use can readily lead to unwanted weight gain. Accordingly, never just sprinkle an oil over foods. Instead, use a spoon to measure out portions (each tablespoon is approximately 120 calories regardless of the type of oil). This will ensure that you get the right amount of fats for optimal bodily function without running the risk of overconsumption.

Remember, for optimizing body composition and overall health, the quality of dietary fat is just as important as the quantity. Approximately 10 percent of intake should come from essential fats, with the ratio of omega-6 to omega-3 fatty acids at about 1:1. When in doubt, err on the side of consuming more omega-3s as they are the most biologically active of all fats. The rest of your consumption should be primarily in the form of MUFAs, with as little saturated and trans fats as possible.

THE BEST SOURCES OF FAT

As discussed, the type of fat you consume is extremely important to body composition and health. Certain foods are rich in the "good" fats and virtually devoid of the "bad" fats, while others have the opposite ratio. Let's take a look at some of the better choices to satisfy your dietary fat requirements.

Nuts

Nuts can be excellent sources of unsaturated fats. They tend to be rich in both MUFAs and PUFAs and are usually low in saturated fats. And as a bonus, they provide fair amounts of protein, fiber, vitamins, and minerals—a nutritional home run.

If possible, choose nuts that are raw and unsalted. Peanut butter should be all natural, without added ingredients. As is true for almost all foods, the less processing and additives, the better.

One of the best things about nuts is that there is a wealth of varieties to choose from, each with its own unique taste and consistency. Good sources of MUFAs include peanuts, pistachios, macadamias, cashews, pecans, and almonds. Walnuts are the one type of nut that has somewhat higher levels of omega-3s, making it a good choice for getting extra PUFAs.

Seeds

Plant seeds are another quality source of unsaturated fats. Depending on the seed, up to 70 percent of the contents are from fat, mostly in the form of MUFAs and PUFAs. And like nuts, seeds also contain healthy amounts of protein, fiber, vitamins, and minerals. Seeds can be chewed whole, making a palatable choice as a snack. Alternatively, they can be ground up and added to your favorite cereals, salads, or just about any other healthy dish you desire.

With their high percentage of omega-3s, flaxseeds are by far the best choice here. Sesame, sunflower, and pumpkin seeds contain mostly omega-6s and therefore should be consumed in moderation to avoid promoting an eicosanoid imbalance.

Fruits and Vegetables

While most people don't think of fruits and vegetables as sources of fat, there are several that fit the bill quite nicely. One of the best is avocados, which are high in MUFAs and low in saturated fats. What's more, they are delicious and can be used in salads, dips, soups, and many other dishes.

Olives are also excellent sources of MUFAs. As with their oil, olives contain predominantly MUFAs and are replete in antioxidants and other healthful compounds. They go great in salads and can be added to a variety of dishes to enhance flavor.

Soybeans are the one vegetable that contains a fair amount of omega-3s (if you remember, they also are a good source of protein). There is some controversy, however, about the long-term health consequences related to soybean consumption and intake should therefore be kept in moderation (see Chapter 5 for recommendations).

Helpful Hint

Unsaturated oils are very susceptible to degradation from light, air, and heat. The more unsaturated the oil, the greater its susceptibility to degradation (i.e., omega-3s are more vulnerable than omega-6s). Once exposed to outside elements for a protracted period of time, the oil becomes rancid, losing most of its healthful properties. To ensure you get the full benefits from an oil, make sure you buy ones that are mechanically (i.e., expeller) pressed under protection from light and air (oils that use this approach state so right on the label) and packaged in an opaque container. Store them in a cool, dry place. Once opened, they should be refrigerated and used within a couple of months.

Oils

Oils are the fats extracted from nuts, seeds, fruits, and vegetables. They can be predominantly saturated (palm oil and coconut oil), monounsaturated (olive and avocado), or polyunsaturated (safflower and flaxseed oil). See Table 6.1 for a dietary breakdown of various oils (note that the data are expressed in percentage of total calories).

As discussed, olive oil is perhaps the best source of MUFAs. When choosing an olive oil, make sure to get one that is "extra virgin." This ensures that it is completely unrefined and hasn't gone through industrial processes like degumming, bleaching, and deodorizing. These procedures remove the health-related benefits of the oil and actually render it harmful to your well-being. I recommend consuming at least one tablespoon of extra virgin olive oil per day. Other good MUFA-based oils include almond and avocado.

For PUFAs, flax oil is the oil of choice. Like the seeds from which it is derived, flax oil contains more than 50 percent omega-3 fatty acids—far more than any other oil. I recommend consuming at least one tablespoon of flax oil per day. Hemp, walnut, and canola oil also have fair amounts of omega-3s, making them good dietary choices.

Oils are extremely versatile foods. Use them on salads, pour them over hot veggies, mix them in with oatmeal and other hot cereals, or add them to a smoothie; the possibilities are virtually endless. Most have a pleasant, nutty taste and can even be taken straight up.

Table 6.1

PERCENTAGE OF DIFFERENT FATS IN VARIOUS OILS				
OIL	**SATURATED**	**OMEGA-9**	**OMEGA-6**	**OMEGA-3**
Almond	9	72	19	None
Avocado	13	72	14	1
Canola	8	60	22	10
Corn	14	26	60	None
Flax	9	16	20	55
Hemp	8	15	56	21
Olive	16	76	8	Trace
Peanut	18	47	35	None
Safflower	10	13	77	Trace
Sesame	15	41	44	Trace
Soybean	15	24	53	8
Sunflower	11	47	42	Trace
Walnut	10	23	56	11

Fish

In addition to being rich in protein, fish also can be excellent sources of essential fats. Because they contain derivatives of omega-3s, namely eicosapentaenoic acid (EPA) and docosahexaenoic acid (DHA), fish oils have even greater utility than high omega-3 foods such as flax. You see, in order for the body to use omega-3s (i.e., alpha-linoleate), it must first *desaturate* them into EPA and DHA. But the desaturation process can be inefficient and potentially result in "lost" nutrients. Since fish oil bypasses this process, there is maximal utilization of the oil.

Realize, though, that not all fish are alike when it comes to containing essential fats. As a rule, the best choices are deep-colored cold-water fish such as salmon, trout, mackerel, and sardines. They are rich in unsaturated fats, with up to 50 percent coming from omega-3s and much of this as preformed EPA and DHA.

For optimal results, aim to eat fish several times a week. This will supplement your consumption of flax oil, ensuring you get enough EPA and DHA. If you can't stomach fish, you can take fish oil capsules; shoot for 5 to 10 grams every other day (each capsule is usually 1 gram).

Summary of the Look Great Naked Diet Guidelines for Dietary Fat

1. Consume a minimum of 15 to 20 percent of calories from fat with total intake based on what remains after adding up calories from carbohydrate and protein.
2. The majority of your fats should be consumed from monounsaturated and polyunsaturated sources.
3. Try to keep the ratio of omega-6 to omega-3 fatty acids close to 1:1 with an emphasis on omega-3s.
4. Limit your intake of saturated and trans fats as much as possible. They are unnecessary and detrimental to your health and wellness.
5. Consume at least one tablespoon of flax oil and one tablespoon of olive oil per day.
6. Eat cold-water fish at least a couple of times a week. If you don't like fish, consider taking supplemental fish oil capsules.

CHAPTER 7

A Thirst for Water

Many people assume that if they pay attention to the carbohydrates, protein, and fat in their diet, they will be covering all the nutritional essentials. Not so. If you're *only* looking at these components of your diet, you're leaving out one of the most important elements—water!

What liquids are you drinking every day? What "good" are they doing your body? And what *should* be your daily intake? If you're going to be successful, your daily water intake can't be left to chance. As you'll see in this chapter, your body depends on water for "detoxification"—that is, to remove and flush out cellular waste products that would otherwise be kidnapped in your tissues. You also need water to help prevent hunger—a key aspect in maintaining dietary adherence—as well as to stave off disease and facilitate cardiovascular health.

I am always surprised when I meet people who cut down on their intake of liquids because they're afraid of "water retention." As you'll see, reducing water intake is decidedly counterproductive. In fact, water deprivation has such a bad effect on the liver that it can actually inhibit its function—and when your liver isn't doing its job, you're likely to store *more* fat rather than less. As for the "bloating" effect that some people get, that's generally associated with too much salt in the diet—not water consumption.

In this chapter, I'll help you determine how much water you need to drink every day to maintain optimum health, keep your energy up, control appetite, flush out metabolic waste, and foster optimum calorie-burning. For many people, the daily intake I recommend is more than the "eight 8-ounce glasses" that has been used as a rule of thumb by many doctors and health experts. On the other hand, you'll discover that the amounts you get from caffeinated beverages and from whole foods like fresh fruit and vegetables can decrease your overall requirements (while the consumption of alcohol will add to it). I'll also suggest some ways to ensure that you're getting as few pollutants as possible in the water that you drink. And you'll learn that, despite the claims of some, there's no need to overload on water. Once you're getting the right amounts, you'll find that any more is superfluous.

REASONS TO DRINK UP

Water is everywhere—at least as far as your body is concerned: Your muscles are roughly 70 percent water; your blood is more than 80 percent water; and your lungs are almost 90 percent water. Water even makes up approximately 25 percent of your bone tissue. That's why it's essential to pay attention to your body's water needs. Many people give little heed to their fluid intake and this lapse in judgment can have far-reaching implications on both your health and body composition.

The consumption of water is integrally involved in maintaining bodily function. It facilitates cells' sending chemical messages to one another, helps to regulate body temperature, and fosters the production and metabolism of energy. Clearly, water is the most vital of all nutrients—without it, you'd die in a matter of days.

But water has numerous benefits over and above the regulation of basic processes. For one, it acts as a detoxifier, assisting the kidneys in cleansing your body of waste products and impurities. This is especially important when you follow a higher protein diet. If you remember, the breakdown of protein results in the production of ammonia, which is then converted to urea. Urea, in turn, must be excreted to avoid negative physiologic complications.

To facilitate the removal of excess urea, your body needs a healthy supply of water.[1] Water helps to flush the kidneys of urea (and other metabolites, as well), allowing them to be safely eliminated in the urine rather than reabsorbed into the body.[2] As long as water intake is sufficient, an increased protein intake poses no problem to your kidneys, liver, or any other internal organ, for that matter.

Water also helps to suppress hunger.[3] Although the exact reasons are unclear, it is theorized that by filling up your stomach, water activates satiety-inducing stretch receptors. The stretch receptors, in turn, send signals back to the brain indicating a sense of fullness. The end result is that you eat less than you otherwise would. Best of all, these satiety-inducing effects are accomplished without adding any calories to your diet (water has no caloric value—no matter how much you consume, it can't increase body fat!).

In addition, water plays a role in disease prevention. Studies show there is a strong dose-dependent relationship between fluid consumption and certain cancers: the more fluids you take in, the lower your chances of getting cancer. For example, the risk of bladder cancer decreases approximately 7 percent for each daily 8-ounce increase in fluid intake.[4] Similar inverse correlations are seen with water consumption and the risk of colorectal cancer and premalignant adenomatous polyps.[5,6,7] And there is some evidence that a link exists between water and reduced rates of breast cancer.

Water consumption is even beneficial to your cardiovascular system. Studies have shown that drinking at least five glasses of water a day can cut the risk of a coronary event by more than 50 percent.[8] It is speculated that water's cardioprotective effects are due to lowering blood viscosity, hematocrit, and fibrinogen, which are considered independent risk factors for coronary heart disease. All things considered, consuming liberal amounts of water is a cheap and easy way to improve your overall wellness.

FLUIDS AND WATER RETENTION

Some people cut back on fluid intake, thinking it will help to eliminate water retention. Women, in particular, subscribe to this misguided practice. Whether it's to counteract the effects of monthly bloating or simply to look better in a bikini, water restriction is an all-too-common practice. Some even go so far as to refrain from drinking liquids altogether, taking their bodies to the point of dehydration.

The truth is, however, limiting water intake is decidedly counterproductive. When fluids are restricted, your body senses a threat to its survival and tries to hold on to every last drop of water. What follows is the classic negative feedback loop. Through a complex series of events, the posterior pituitary gland is signaled to secrete antidiuretic hormone (ADH).[9] ADH acts on the kidneys, causing them to reduce their output of urine and reabsorb fluids back into circulation. The end result is an increase in water retention, leaving you puffy and bloated.[10]

Without an adequate supply of water, your kidneys start to "back up," causing a systemic accumulation of metabolic waste.[11] Consequently, your liver has to work overtime to neutralize these waste products. This compromises your liver's ability to metabolize fat into usable energy—one of its primary responsibilities. As a result, less fat is burned for fuel, heightening the potential for increased fat storage.

The real culprit in water retention is sodium intake—most commonly consumed as salt in the diet. Because it carries an electrical charge, sodium is considered an *electrolyte*. In conjunction with potassium, it is responsible for regulating the body's fluid balance; potassium maintains the fluid balance *intracellularly* (within the cells), while sodium maintains the balance of fluids *extracellularly* (outside of the cells). Hence, sodium is essential for bodily function; a lack of it leads to *hyponatremia*, a condition that, when severe, ultimately causes death.

But although it is an essential nutrient, only minute quantities of sodium are required through dietary means. In fact, a mere 500 milligrams is all that's needed to maintain normal biologic function—an amount that equates to about a ¼ of a teaspoon of salt.[12] Yet the average American consumes more than ten times this quantity! When too much sodium is ingested, fluid is drawn out of the cells and into the interstitial spaces, causing the body to retain water.[13]

So, to reduce bloating, drink plenty of water and try cutting back on salty foods. In order to avoid any hidden sources of sodium, get used to reading food labels. The sodium content is plainly listed for all to see. And don't worry about a deficiency: sodium occurs naturally in most foods and you'll get all you need just by eating a sensible diet. Remember, restricting fluid intake is decidedly disadvantageous, not only to body composition, but also to overall health. It causes diminished water excretion and actually causes your body to retain water.

Helpful Hint

The best way to avoid ingesting too much sodium is by eating fresh, unprocessed foods. Stay away from all prepackaged and canned goods; they tend to be loaded with sodium. So are many condiments; ketchup, salad dressings, and soy sauce all contain whopping amounts.

In addition, refrain from adding salt to your meals. If you want to spice up your foods, there are dozens of delicious seasonings that can enhance flavor without negative complications. Paprika, cinnamon, basil, oregano, garlic—the list is almost endless. Experiment with different combinations and see what you find palatable. By using a little ingenuity, you can create tasty dishes that are virtually sodium-free.

HOW MUCH DO YOU NEED?

Although the importance of consuming ample amounts of fluids is well documented, there is a paucity of scientific data as to exactly what constitutes an optimal intake. Since average water losses amount to just a little more than a quart per day, you really don't need to consume much to offset what you use up.[14] But simply replacing what is lost isn't enough to keep your body running at peak efficiency.

A common prescription is to drink eight 8-ounce glasses a day—the so-called 8 × 8 rule. However, this formula doesn't take into account differences in body size, and there's little doubt that a burly guy needs more fluids than a petite woman. A good rule of thumb is to take in at least a half ounce of water per pound of ideal body weight, spacing out intake throughout the day. Thus, a person who wants to weigh 150 pounds should consume approximately 75 ounces of water. Whenever possible, water should be chilled or served on ice. Cold water is absorbed into the system more quickly than warm water, ensuring a continued state of hydration.

Part of your daily fluid needs will also be furnished by the foods you eat. It's estimated that the typical diet supplies about 35 ounces of water.[15] Carbohydrates—particularly fresh fruits and vegetables—contain large quantities of water, as do most proteins and fats. So when figuring out your requirements, subtract about a quart (32 ounces) of fluids from the total.

> Water consumption = ½ ounce water × ideal body weight − 32 ounces

Contrary to popular belief, caffeine-based beverages count toward meeting your daily fluid needs. Although they exert a mild diuretic effect, the majority of liquid in caffeinated drinks is retained by your body.[16] So whether you enjoy coffee, tea, or colas (diet, of course!), drinking beverages that contain caffeine will help to keep you hydrated.

Alcohol is another story. It has a significant diuretic effect—so significant, in fact, that it can actually exacerbate dehydration when consumed in large quantities.[17] The reasons are twofold: First, alcohol inhibits the release of antidiuretic hormone (ADH).[18] This promotes excessive urination, causing your body to deplete its water stores. What's more, the metabolism of alcohol is an energy-intensive process; a good deal of water is used up in its breakdown. So when you consume an alcoholic beverage, you end up losing about as much water as you gain from the drink itself.

As an aside, it is unnecessary and perhaps counterproductive to take in massive quantities of fluids. Doing so can result in water intoxication, a condition that disrupts nerve cell function.[19] Although rare (most people are able to excrete excess water within a wide range of intake), this condition can affect young and old alike with potentially serious complications from disoriented behavior to convulsions, coma, and death. Just stick to the suggested guidelines and you'll have all the water you need for a terrific body.

WHAT TO DRINK

Believe it or not, there is a difference in water quality. All water is not alike and the type you choose can have an impact on health and wellness. As a rule, try to avoid regular tap water. Despite the purification attempts by government municipalities, it is filled with contaminants that can have an adverse effect on your body. Chlorine and fluoride, in particular, have been implicated in a variety of health problems, including cancer and birth defects.[20,21,22] Trace amounts of radon, lead, arsenic, and other undesirable elements have also been observed in water drawn from our reservoirs.[23]

If you must drink from the sink, your best bet is to get a filtering system. This helps to purify water and make it more fit for human consumption. Boiling tap water aids in destroying disease-causing bacteria, viruses, and related microorganisms. It will not, however, remove nitrates, pesticides, and other inorganic chemicals from water and can actually increase the concentration of these contaminants.

A better alternative is to drink natural spring water. Generally speaking, spring water is devoid of the pollutants that taint our reservoirs and therefore keeps your body free of contaminants.[24] Make sure to get a brand from a reputable bottling company, though. If quality control is poor, springs can become tainted and, in some cases, contain as many or more toxins than what is found in reservoirs.[25,26]

Summary of the Look Great Naked Diet Water Protocol

1. Consume roughly a half ounce of water per pound of ideal body weight, minus one quart (the amount of water you get from your diet).
2. Caffeinated beverages count toward daily requirements; alcohol does not.
3. There is no need to overload on water and it potentially can have negative effects on your health.
4. To avoid contaminants, drink bottled water whenever possible. Alternatively, get a filtering system for your tap.

THE LGN
PROGRAM

PART THREE

CHAPTER 8

A Body to Diet For

By now, you should have a firm grasp of nutritional basics. This knowledge will be indispensable in developing a personalized nutritional approach; one that is tailored to your individual situation. But while knowledge is power, it's the application of knowledge that breeds results.

Optimal body composition is achieved only by properly manipulating the amounts, types, and ratios of the foods that you eat in accordance with your individual needs and goals. Suffice it to say, the extent to which you get these variables right will ultimately determine your success in attaining the physique you desire.

CALORIES COUNT

As previously stated, energy balance is the overriding determinant in long-term weight management: If calorie consumption is more than what you expend, you'll gain weight; if calorie consumption is less than what you expend, you'll lose weight;

Daily Caloric Maintenance Level

Men	Women
DCML = Body weight × 15	DCML = Body weight × 14

and if calorie consumption is equal to what you expend, you'll maintain your weight. This is the basis of the laws of thermodynamics, and for all intents and purposes, the laws are immutable.

The fact is, however, dieters tend to place far too much emphasis on what they eat at the expense of how much they eat—a philosophy that is destined for failure. You can consume all the "right" foods, but if you take in too many calories from these foods, weight gain is inevitable. Hypothetically, consuming 2,000 calories of broccoli will make you fat if your daily expenditure is only 1,500 calories (although it would be next to impossible to consume the 20-plus pounds of broccoli required to reach this level of caloric intake). It is therefore essential that you get a firm hold on how many calories you take in. Consuming as few as an extra 100 calories a day— the amount found in a handful of nachos or a dozen French fries—can result in a yearly weight gain of more than 10 pounds!

In order to determine how many calories you should consume, you must first figure out your daily caloric maintenance level (DCML): the number of calories required each day to maintain a stable body weight. A simple way to estimate DCML is by using a body-weight multiplier (keep in mind that protein and carbs have four calories per gram and fat has nine calories per gram). The body-weight multiplier is based on target body weight and is gender specific: Men should multiply their target body weight by 15; women should multiply their target body weight by 14. Thus, a man who wants to weigh 200 pounds would have a DCML of about 3,000 calories while a woman who wants to weigh 125 pounds would have a DCML of approximately 1,750 calories.

Understand that the body-weight multiplier formula provides only a crude approximation of daily caloric intake. Many things influence actual caloric requirements, including activity levels, hormonal production, non-exercise activity thermogenesis (i.e., fidgeting), the thermic effect of food, and others. You should use the DCML as a starting point from which to work. Over time, modifications can be made based on individual requirements.

In order to get a handle on portions, it can be beneficial to weigh your foods, at least during the beginning stages of your diet. Make an investment in a digital food scale. They are fairly inexpensive (a good one can cost less than $50) and extremely accurate. Once you've weighed the foods for a period of time, portions will become instinctive: You'll know what a 4-ounce chicken breast looks like; you'll be able to eyeball a cup of rice without a measuring cup.

If you don't want to go through the hassle of weighing foods, that's fine. Just make sure you aren't overdoing it with your portions. Eat too much and you will gain body fat, regardless of the composition of nutrients.

GET YOUR TYPES RIGHT

The importance of portion control doesn't mean that the kind of foods you eat is irrelevant. On the contrary, all calories are *not* created equal and the types and ratios of foods in your diet most certainly will have an effect on body composition. As previously discussed, certain foods are more metabolic than others. Due to their effects on thermogenesis, hormones, enzymes, and other factors, foods have both a direct and indirect impact on what is stored and what is burned. This not only applies to the individual macronutrient ratios of carbs, protein, fat, and water, but also to different types of the same macronutrient (e.g., saturated, monounsaturated, and polyunsaturated fats).

Just to review the basics:

- Carbohydrate intake should be based on your body type.
- Consumption of carbohydrates and fats should maintain an inverse relationship; the more carbs in your diet, the less fat and vice versa.
- Regardless of how many calories you consume, protein intake should always be a constant, amounting to one gram of protein per pound of goal body weight.

As with DCML, your exact macronutrient ratios will probably need to be adapted somewhat as you go along. While most people should only have to make minor adjustments, individual variations can occasionally require somewhat larger than expected deviations. Just be in tune with your body and don't be afraid to experiment until you get it right.

MONITORING PROGRESS

Your progress should be monitored on a regular basis. For most, the scale is the measurement tool of choice. A word of caution, though: Don't become scale obsessed! When a person begins a weight-loss program, there is a tendency to rely on the scale as their "report card." Women, in particular, tend to fall into this rut. They'll weigh themselves several times a day, freaking out whenever they gain a pound. This can end up being a real de-motivator.

Realize that the scale doesn't distinguish between body fat, lean tissue, and water weight. It simply measures overall body mass. This is especially problematic for premenopausal women, where the menstrual cycle creates hormonal ebbs and flows that result in brief periods of water retention. And although water has no bearing on body fat percentage, it does register on the scale as weight gain.

If you work out (as you certainly should!), the scale is even more of an enigma. Muscle is much denser than fat and consequently weighs more by volume. A golf ball, for example, weighs more than a tennis ball even though it is much smaller in overall diameter. So adding muscle can actually "redistribute" your proportions. You might be a little heavier on the scale, but you'll have lower body-fat levels and look better in or out of clothes. Remember, weight is only a number and the most important thing is how you look and feel, not how much you weigh.

That said, the scale can be a convenient way to assess how you're doing. If you want to weigh yourself, do so first thing in the morning, before you've had anything to eat. And make sure you use the same scale each time (preferably one that is not used by multiple people). This will minimize the potential for variation, ensuring the most consistent readings possible.

A better alternative to the scale is body-fat testing. Because it distinguishes between fat and lean tissue, body-fat testing gives a much more realistic picture of your actual body composition. The most common technique is the skin-fold method, where a calipers is used to take measurements from select areas on your body. Most personal trainers will be able to do this at your local gym. Just make sure the trainer has experience in testing. When not done properly, measurements can be way off (and I've seen a lot of whacky percentages quoted!).

GO FOR THE GOAL

What follows are detailed strategies for realizing various physique goals. Provided you adhere to the guidelines as directed, the possibilities for redefining your body are almost limitless within your own genetic framework.

GOAL: LOSE BODY FAT

Given that a majority of the population is overweight, it should come as no surprise that the goal of most people is to lose body fat. Unfortunately, a significant portion of people often resort to using extreme diets in an attempt to slim down as quickly as possible. Our society craves instant gratification and the prospect of a rapid physical transformation is hard to resist. After all, who doesn't want to leave work on a Friday and come back Monday morning looking like a new person?

The truth is, however, extreme diets don't work—at least over the long haul. One of the biggest problems with these diets is that they not only reduce fat, but they catabolize lean tissue, too. When calories are severely restricted, up to 45 percent of the energy deficit is derived from burning muscle for fuel—a fact that can account for as much as one pound a week of muscle loss.[1] Since muscle tissue is metabolically active, its loss causes an associated drop in metabolic rate. The combination of these factors makes it increasingly more difficult to shed unwanted pounds and, in the end, regained weight is almost always higher than it was before dieting.[2]

Extreme dieting also has a negative effect on leptin. Levels of the hormone fall dramatically, far above the actual amount of weight loss. This disproportionate drop in leptin sets into motion a neurochemical cascade that sets off wild hunger cravings, a fall in metabolic rate, and an increase in the activity of the fat-storing enzyme lipoprotein lipase.[3]

On top of everything, extreme dieting also has a negative impact on thyroid function. Specifically, it results in both a reduced synthesis of T3 (triiodothyronine, the active thyroid hormone) as well as a decrease in the number of active thyroid receptors.[4] Since T3 is a potent thermogenic agent, these events put the brakes on metabolic rate[5] (especially in combination with decreased leptin production). Ultimately, your metabolism slows to a crawl, making a return to set point inevitable. This creates a vicious cycle where calories must be continually decreased in order to sustain weight loss. After a while, a point of diminishing returns is reached and the body simply becomes resistant to any more weight loss. Inevitably, when the diet is discontinued, body weight balloons back up—often in excess of the original starting point.

The worst thing you can do is go through repeated cycles of weight loss and regain (called yo-yo dieting) as this can have long-term effects on suppressing metabolism.[6,7,8] During each diet cycle, the body continually trains itself to survive on fewer and fewer calories. In an attempt to maintain homeostasis, it alters various hormonal and enzymatic mechanisms, and, in certain cases, these alterations can be difficult to reverse. Inevitably, set point goes up and there is a predisposition to retaining body fat in later cycles[9] (the classic rebound effect).

Determining Calorie Intake

Instead of going for a quick fix, you need to take a practical approach to shedding unwanted body fat. To this end, a maximum of one to two pounds can be lost per week. Any more and you'll not only lose fat, but you'll simultaneously lose lean muscle tissue—a surefire ticket to a sluggish metabolism. While a loss of one pound of fat per week might not seem like a lot on the surface, over the course of a year it equates to a 50-pound drop! As they say, patience is a virtue and provided you stay the course, you'll be aptly rewarded with a terrific physique.

To effectively lose fat, your DCML must be adjusted so you expend more calories than you consume. Initially, you should aim for a 500 calorie a day reduction. For example, a woman who wants to weigh 125 pounds would have a daily caloric requirement of approximately 1,250 calories (i.e., $125 \times 14 = 1,750 - 500 = 1,250$). In most cases, this should be sufficient to achieve desired results.

If, over time, you are not losing weight as desired, you should increase the caloric deficit to 600 calories a day and see how you do at this level. Continue the reassessment process on a regular basis, adjusting intake as needed. But don't go overboard. Losing too much, too soon is bound to sabotage your long-term physique goals.

Regardless of your DCML, don't go below about 1,000 calories a day. This represents a bare minimum to meet your daily nutrient needs and prevent the breakdown of muscle tissue. Remember, with respect to weight loss, less can be more.

Also, keep in mind that weight loss is not always linear. Rather, it tends to be like a roller coaster, with numerous peaks and valleys. Some weeks you might lose several pounds while others you might stay the same or even gain a pound or two (as discussed, this is especially the case in premenopausal women). Just maintain perspective and things will work out for the best.

The Refeed Day

To maximize fat loss, you should employ a regularly scheduled "refeed" day. Think of the refeed as a holiday from your diet, where you can eat virtually anything you want, including sugar and/or fat-laden foods. Within reason, there are no restrictions. Go ahead and order a pizza. Frequent your favorite fast-food restaurant. Have a candy bar. Whatever you heart desires, feel free to indulge.

The refeed day serves a dual purpose. For one, it helps you keep your sanity. The biggest diet-related fear of most people is that they'll have to adhere to a strict nutritional regimen forever, and the thought of never again enjoying their favorite foods is often too much to bear. After several months of deprivation, they break down and go on an eating binge, scoffing down everything in sight. At that point, the diet goes out the window.

By providing a weekly respite from your diet, the refeed day allows you to satisfy all your cravings. In this way, you won't feel food deprived, making dieting a much more favorable experience. And when you are content with your diet, there's less of a tendency to binge, translating into better results.

In addition to the psychological boost provided by the refeed, there also are distinct physiological benefits. Specifically, it has a positive influence on leptin levels, with results seen immediately after refeeding.[10,11] Although the primary function of leptin is to control long-term maintenance of body-fat levels, it also plays a role in monitoring short-term changes in food consumption.[12,13] While leptin doesn't by itself lead to termination of a meal, it does function locally in the stomach, increasing during periods of overfeeding and decreasing during periods of underfeeding.[14] By upping food intake every so often, you "trick" your body into thinking it isn't under calorie restriction, thereby mitigating any drop in leptin production.[15,16,17]

To heighten the beneficial effects on leptin, it's advisable to eat a good portion of calories from carb-based foods (particularly non-fibrous starches) during the refeed. Glucose, the constituent of starch, increases leptin production much more so than fatty foods.[18] Pasta, rice, breads, and other starches make excellent choices for refeed. Even simple sugars such as cookies and cakes are fine. It's one of the few times that high-glycemic foods are actually desirable.

While you are free to eat your favorite foods, it is important not to binge on the refeed day. Ideally, you should keep the total calories on your refeed to about 150 percent of your DCML. For instance, if your DCML is 2,000 calories, don't go past 3,000 calories or so. This will give you plenty of leeway to satisfy your cravings and rev up leptin production while still keeping caloric intake within a reasonable range. Although a little bit of planned overindulgence is desirable, consuming mass quantities of food is likely to impair body composition (as well as making you pretty sick!).

It is important that your refeed day be a regimented affair. Don't let cheating become a habit. Stick with the program as directed and make your refeed a planned event. In this way, you don't have to feel guilty about eating your favorite foods; consider it a reward for sticking to your diet.

Customizing a Fat-Loss Diet

What follows is the three-step process for customizing a fat-loss diet. For illustrative purposes, we will use the example of a female Type I (see Chapter 4) with a target body weight of 125 pounds. Based on DCML, total estimated caloric intake will be 1,250 calories (i.e., $125 \times 14 = 1,750 - 500 = 1,250$).

STEP ONE: DETERMINE PROTEIN INTAKE

This number will be fixed regardless of how many calories you consume. Remember that protein intake corresponds to one gram per pound of goal body weight. Because protein has 4 calories per gram, to determine how many calories of protein to consume, multiply your protein intake in grams by 4. So for our example, total daily protein consumption will amount to 500 calories (i.e., 125 grams × 4 calories per gram = 500 calories).

STEP TWO: DETERMINE CARBOHYDRATE INTAKE

The Type I, as discussed in Chapter 4, generally does best on a lower-carb diet corresponding to approximately 35 to 40 percent of total calories. To minimize the potential for fat deposition, it's generally best to start out on the low end of the recommended carb ratio so we'll go with 35 percent. Hence, we multiply total calories by 35 percent and come up with 438 calories of carbs (i.e., .35 × 1,250 total calories = 438). Since each gram of carbs is 4 calories, you'll consume approximately 109 grams of carbs.

STEP THREE: DETERMINE FAT INTAKE

Calories from fat are what's left over after total calories from protein and carbs are subtracted from your estimated caloric intake. Since protein amounts to 500 calories and carbs are 438 calories, fat will be 312 calories (1,250 total calories minus 938 calories from protein and carbs = 312 calories). And since each gram of fat is 9 calories, 35 grams will come from dietary fat.

In this example, you'd have a diet consisting of 35 percent carbohydrate (131 grams), 40 percent protein (125 grams), and 25 percent fat (35 grams). The following is a seven-day sample meal plan that illustrates the concepts of a fat-loss diet. As in the previous example, caloric intake is estimated at 1,250 calories. Of course, you will need to adjust the amount of calories based on your individual needs.

Day One

MEAL ONE
- 2 slices multigrain bread
- Mushroom omelet (6 egg whites and 1 portobello mushroom)
- 1 tablespoon flaxseed oil
- 1 or 2 cups coffee or tea

MEAL TWO
- 1 large plum

MEAL THREE
- Tuna salad (6 ounces of tuna, mixed greens, and 1 tablespoon olive oil)
- 1 medium sweet potato

MEAL FOUR
- 1 medium pear

MEAL FIVE
- 4 ounces turkey breast
- 12 ounces cauliflower

Day Two

MEAL ONE
- 6 ounces cottage cheese (99 percent fat-free)
- 2 slices multigrain bread
- 1 or 2 cups coffee or tea

MEAL TWO
- 1 large orange

MEAL THREE
- 4 ounces tofu
- Large salad (romaine lettuce, green pepper, carrot, tomato, onion, balsamic vinegar, and 1 tablespoon olive oil)

MEAL FOUR
- Blueberry smoothie (1 cup blueberries, 1 scoop whey protein powder, 1 tablespoon flaxseed oil, and crushed ice)

MEAL FIVE
- 6 ounces Chilean sea bass
- 12 ounces snap green beans

Day Three

MEAL ONE
- 1 cup cream of wheat
- 1 tablespoon flaxseed oil

- 1 scoop whey protein powder
- 1 or 2 cups coffee or tea

MEAL TWO
- 1 cup strawberries

MEAL THREE
- 4 ounces chicken breast
- ½ cup brown rice

MEAL FOUR
- 1 cup plain yogurt

MEAL FIVE
- 4 ounces sirloin steak
- 12 ounces asparagus
- 1 tablespoon olive oil

Day Four

MEAL ONE
- ½ cup oatmeal
- 1 scoop whey protein powder
- 1 tablespoon flaxseed oil
- 1 or 2 cups coffee or tea

MEAL TWO
- 1 ounce seedless raisins

MEAL THREE
- Chicken sandwich (4 ounces sliced chicken breast on rye bread)
- Large salad (romaine lettuce, green pepper, carrot, tomato, onion, balsamic vinegar, and 1 tablespoon olive oil)

MEAL FOUR
- 1 cup cubed honeydew melon

MEAL FIVE
- 6 ounces shrimp
- 12 ounces spinach

Day Five

MEAL ONE
- 1 cup shredded wheat
- 4 ounces milk (99 percent fat-free)
- 1 or 2 cups coffee or tea

MEAL TWO
- Banana smoothie (1 large banana, 1 scoop whey protein powder, 1 tablespoon flaxseed oil, and crushed ice)

MEAL THREE
- 6 ounces Cornish game hen breast
- Large salad (romaine lettuce, green pepper, carrot, tomato, onion, balsamic vinegar, and 1 tablespoon olive oil)

MEAL FOUR
- 1 large peach

MEAL FIVE
- 6 ounces orange roughy
- 12 ounces zucchini

Day Six

MEAL ONE
- 1 cup all-bran cereal
- 4 ounces milk (99 percent fat-free)
- 1 or 2 cups coffee or tea

MEAL TWO
- 1 medium mango

MEAL THREE
- Turkey sandwich (4 ounces sliced turkey breast on whole-wheat bread)
- Large salad (romaine lettuce, green pepper, carrot, tomato, onion, balsamic vinegar, and 1 tablespoon olive oil)

MEAL FOUR
- 1 cup plain yogurt
- 1 tablespoon flaxseed oil

MEAL FIVE
- 6 ounces fillet of sole
- 12 ounces broccoli

Day Seven: Refeed Day
(about 2,500 calories)

MEAL ONE
- Pancakes with maple syrup

MEAL TWO
- 1 jelly doughnut

MEAL THREE
- Cheeseburger with lettuce and tomato on sesame seed bun

MEAL FOUR
- 1 cup cookies-'n'-cream ice cream

MEAL FIVE
- 2 slices cheese pizza

GOAL: BULKING UP

The thought of eating to *gain* weight is completely foreign to many people. In fact, with so many struggling to keep their weight down, some would go so far as to call it heresy. But certain individuals, especially "pure" Type IIIs, have a difficult time bulking up. This is exemplified by the prototypical 90-pound weakling who regards being skinny as a curse. As depicted in the comics, it's not much fun to get sand kicked in your face at the beach!

It should be noted that adding mass isn't exclusively a concern of Type IIIs. Bodybuilders, football players, and other strength athletes all share the same goal of seeking to bulk up at specific times during their competitive cycles. For these individuals, maximizing muscle mass is essential to achieving aesthetic balance and enhancing physical performance.

In truth, anyone can put on weight provided they consume enough calories. Even the scrawniest Type III will eventually get beefier by scoffing down tons of cheeseburgers, fries, and milk shakes.[19] The problem with such a strategy is that far too much of the gains will be in the form of body fat. Consequently, the weight invariably ends up being distributed in all the wrong places, creating a "skinny-flabby" appearance.

Moreover, gaining a large amount of body fat is harmful over the long term. Remember, when fat cells reach a certain size, they undergo hyperplasia and split into more fat cells. And once new adipocytes are formed, you can't get rid of them. This raises set point, making it more difficult to retain a lean appearance in the future.

The best way to go about bulking up is by adding quality weight, meaning the weight is in the form of lean muscle tissue—not body fat. To this end, it is essential that you refrain from bulking up too rapidly. A gain of about one pound per week is the upper limit of what you can expect to attain without significantly increasing body-fat levels.

To accomplish this task, your DCML must be adjusted so you consume more calories than you expend. Generally, it is best to aim for a caloric surplus of 500 calories a day. For example, a guy who wants to weigh 175 pounds would have a daily caloric requirement of approximately 3,125 calories (i.e., $175 \times 15 = 2,625 + 500 = 3,125$).

If, over time, you aren't gaining enough mass, increase daily intake by 100 calories (i.e., you would now consume an extra 600 calories a day). Alternatively, if you are gaining too much fat for your liking, cut back by 100 calories (i.e., to a 400 calorie surplus) and, if necessary, reduce carbs and increase unsaturated fats. Making these adjustments in a controlled, systematic fashion will allow you to fine-tune your diet so optimal results are achieved.

Unfortunately, set point will often get in the way of your mass-gaining efforts. As previously discussed, set point not only works to prevent attempts at weight loss, but also at weight gain. When you put on weight, leptin and other satiety systems signal the brain to speed up metabolism and decrease the urge to eat. This makes it difficult to take in the required amount of calories to achieve further gains in mass, especially if your genetics aren't suited to bulking up.

To counter these events, carb intake can be a little on the high side here, with more "white" starches and simple sugars included in your diet (especially for real hardgainers). This serves a dual purpose. For one, high-glycemic carbs trigger hunger mechanisms, stimulating the urge to eat. What's more, the associated increased insulin response helps to increase protein synthesis, promoting the accretion of lean muscle mass.

Given the higher carb intake, the amount of fat in a mass-building diet will necessarily be lower. This is important because when a surplus of calories is consumed, those coming from fat are more easily converted to fat tissue. Excess fat calories have a conversion efficiency of around 98 percent, while the conversion efficiency for carbs is only about 70 percent.[20]

You also might want to take in a greater percentage of calories in liquid form. Since liquids quickly pass through your system, they bypass usual hunger mechanisms, allowing you to consume more quality food. Fruit juices are fine, provided they are consumed in moderation. Remember that the body has only a limited capacity to process fructose (the primary fruit sugar)—any excess is preferentially stored as fat.

If you prefer, there are many weight-gain shakes available to facilitate your bulking efforts. Look for one that's low in fat (especially saturated fat) and higher in carbs and protein. This will provide an anabolic thrust, heightening muscle protein synthesis. Of course, taste is a big issue, too. You really need to *enjoy* your meals to successfully gain mass, and if your shake tastes like paste, your appetite is bound to suffer. So try out a few brands with the suggested profiles and go with the one you like best.

For optimal results, it's imperative that you combine the diet with regimented strength training. Without exercise, approximately 75 percent of weight gain is deposited in the form of fat.[21] Even under the best-case scenario, results will be subpar if you don't work out.

In the initial stages of training, you can simultaneously gain lean tissue while losing body fat. However, after a year or two of working out, doing so becomes increasingly difficult. So for those who are advanced exercisers, the ultimate objective of a mass-gaining regimen should be to maximize the accretion of lean tissue while minimizing fat deposition.

Customizing a Mass-Building Diet

What follows is the three-step process for customizing a mass-building diet. For illustrative purposes, we will use the example of a male Type III with a target body weight of 200 pounds. Based on DCML, total estimated caloric intake will be 3,500 calories (i.e., $200 \times 15 = 3,000 + 500 = 3,500$).

STEP ONE: DETERMINE PROTEIN INTAKE

This number will be fixed regardless of how many calories you consume. Since protein intake corresponds to one gram per pound of goal body weight, total daily protein consumption will amount to 800 calories (i.e., 200 grams $\times$ 4 calories per gram = 800 calories).

STEP TWO: DETERMINE CARBOHYDRATE INTAKE

Type IIIs (see Chapter 4) generally do best on a higher carb diet corresponding to approximately 55 to 60 percent of total calories. To minimize the potential for fat deposition, we'll start out on the lower end of the spectrum at 55 percent. Hence, we multiply total calories by 55 percent and come up with 1,925 calories of carbs (i.e., .55 × 3,500 total calories = 1,925). Since each gram of carbs is four calories, you'll consume approximately 481 grams of carbs.

STEP THREE: DETERMINE FAT INTAKE

Calories from fat are what's left over after total calories from protein and carbs are subtracted from your estimated caloric intake. Since protein amounts to 800 calories and carbs are 1,925 calories, fat will be 775 calories (3,500 total calories minus 2,725 calories from protein and carbs = 775 calories). As each gram of fat is nine calories, approximately 86 grams will come from dietary fat.

Putting it all together, you'd have a diet consisting of 55 percent carbohydrate (481 grams), 23 percent protein (200 grams), and 22 percent fat (86 grams).

The following is a seven-day sample meal plan that illustrates the concepts of a bulking-up diet. As in the previous example, caloric intake is estimated at 3,500 calories. Of course, you will need to adjust the amount of calories based on your individual needs.

Day One

MEAL ONE
- 1 large sesame seed bagel
- Vegetable egg white omelet (6 egg whites, mushrooms, green peppers, and onions)
- 12 ounces orange juice
- 1 or 2 cups coffee or tea

MEAL TWO
- Blackberry smoothie (1 cup blackberries, 1 scoop whey protein powder, 1 tablespoon flaxseed oil, and crushed ice)

MEAL THREE
- Tuna salad (6 ounces tuna, arugula, tomato, and 1 tablespoon olive oil)
- 8 ounces angel hair pasta

MEAL FOUR

- 6 ounces chicken breast
- 2 cups long-grain white rice
- 1 large pear

MEAL FIVE

- 6 ounces sirloin steak
- 2 large sweet potatoes
- 8 ounces cauliflower

Day Two

MEAL ONE

- 1 cup oatmeal
- 2 ounces raisins
- 12 ounces milk (98 percent fat-free)
- 1 scoop whey protein powder
- 1 or 2 cups coffee or tea

MEAL TWO

- Weight-gain shake (100 grams carbohydrate and 50 grams protein)
- 1 tablespoon flaxseed oil

MEAL THREE

- Turkey sandwich (8 ounces turkey breast on whole-wheat pita bread)
- Large avocado salad (1 medium avocado, arugula, green pepper, carrot, tomato, balsamic vinegar, and 1 tablespoon olive oil)
- 12 ounces cranberry juice

MEAL FOUR

- 2 cups brown rice
- 1 cup black beans
- 1 large apple

MEAL FIVE

- 16 ounces low-fat zucchini lasagna

Day Three

MEAL ONE
- 4 large Belgian waffles with maple syrup
- 1 tablespoon flaxseed oil
- 12 ounces pink grapefruit juice
- 1 or 2 cups coffee or tea

MEAL TWO
- Chicken salad (6-ounce chicken breast, romaine lettuce, green pepper, carrot, tomato, balsamic vinegar, and 1 tablespoon olive oil)
- 8 ounces whole-wheat pasta

MEAL THREE
- Steak sandwich (8-ounce sirloin strip steak and 2 slices rye bread)
- 16 ounces mixed fruit salad

MEAL FOUR
- 4 ounces couscous
- 4 ounces black beans

MEAL FIVE
- 6 ounces salmon
- 2 large yams
- 8 ounces collard greens

Day Four

MEAL ONE
- 1 large pumpernickel bagel
- 4 ounces cottage cheese (98 percent fat-free)
- 12 ounces orange juice
- 1 or 2 cups coffee or tea

MEAL TWO
- Tuna salad (6 ounces tuna, arugula, tomato, and 1 tablespoon olive oil)
- 2 cups brown rice

MEAL THREE
- Macaroni and cheese (8 ounces macaroni, 1 cup 98 percent fat-free milk, 6 ounces fat-free cheddar cheese, and 2 whole eggs)

MEAL FOUR
- Ham sandwich (4 ounces ham and 2 slices multigrain bread)
- 1 large peach

MEAL FIVE
- 6 ounces trout
- 2 large sweet potatoes
- 8 ounces green beans

Day Five

MEAL ONE
- 1 cup Grape-Nuts cereal
- 1 cup milk (98 percent fat-free)
- 1 or 2 cups coffee or tea

MEAL TWO
- Weight-gain shake (100 grams carbohydrate and 50 grams protein)
- 1 tablespoon flaxseed oil

MEAL THREE
- 8 ounces whole-wheat linguine
- 1 cup clams
- 1 large banana

MEAL FOUR
- 6 ounces turkey breast
- 1 cup brown rice
- Large salad (romaine lettuce, green pepper, carrot, tomato, onion, balsamic vinegar, and 1 tablespoon olive oil)

MEAL FIVE
- 6 ounces filet mignon
- 12 ounces green peas

Day Six

MEAL ONE
- Mushroom omelet (6 egg whites and 1 portobello mushroom)
- 4 slices multigrain bread
- 12 ounces pineapple juice
- 1 or 2 cups coffee or tea

MEAL TWO
- Strawberry smoothie (1 cup strawberries, 1 scoop whey protein powder, 1 tablespoon flaxseed oil, and crushed ice)

MEAL THREE
- Soy burger (12-ounce soy patty on large poppy seed bagel)
- Large salad (romaine lettuce, green pepper, carrot, tomato, onion, balsamic vinegar, and 1 tablespoon olive oil)

MEAL FOUR
- 8 ounces whole-wheat spaghetti
- 6 ounces turkey breast
- 1 large pear

MEAL FIVE
- 6 ounces mackerel
- 1 cup brown rice
- 8 ounces spinach

Day Seven

MEAL ONE
- 6 large pancakes with maple syrup
- 12 ounces apple juice
- 1 or 2 cups coffee or tea

MEAL TWO
- Weight-gain shake (100 grams carbohydrate and 50 grams protein)
- 1 tablespoon flaxseed oil

MEAL THREE
- 12 ounces cheese tortellini
- Large salad (romaine lettuce, green pepper, carrot, tomato, onion, balsamic vinegar, and 1 tablespoon olive oil)

MEAL FOUR
- 8-ounce chicken breast
- 1 yam
- 1 cup strawberries

MEAL FIVE
- 12 ounces striped bass
- 1 cup brown rice
- 8 ounces asparagus

GOAL: WEIGHT MAINTENANCE

For those fortunate enough to have attained their ideal body composition, a maintenance strategy is in order. Maintenance involves keeping caloric intake in balance with caloric expenditure. Thus, the amount of calories you consume will be the same as your DCML. To review, this number is derived by multiplying your current weight by 14 if you're a woman or 15 if you're a man. Of course, DCML is only an estimate and some degree of adjustment in total calories might be necessary to reflect your new set point.

If you are coming off a fat-loss or mass-gaining diet, it is best to reduce or increase calories incrementally until you reach maintenance level. This allows your body to slowly acclimate to the new caloric level and prevent any reactive hormonal fluctuations from interfering with metabolism and/or appetite. What's more, you can more readily see how your body responds to the new caloric level and make adjustments on the fly. For instance, if you have been dieting to lose weight, add back 100 calories a week until you reach your DCML. On the other hand, if you've been on a mass-building diet, subtract 100 calories a week. Either way, you'll be at maintenance level within a short period of time.

An effective strategy for keeping set point elevated over time is to stagger caloric intake. In this way, you intersperse high-calorie days with low-calorie days, thereby tricking your body into thinking food is abundant. I've found that a three-day rotation of 500 calorie increments works very well. For example, if your DCML is 2,000 calories, you might consume 1,500 calories on day one, 2,000 on day two, and 2,500 on day three. Of course, many other permutations are possible so don't hesitate to experiment and find what works best within the context of your lifestyle.

At this point, the refeed day shouldn't be necessary for sustaining leptin levels (since leptin levels should be regulated to your new set point). However, if you want to have a cheat day for psychological reasons, you certainly are entitled to it. If you choose to indulge in a cheat day, you must reduce calories on your "non-cheat" days accordingly. Remember that weight maintenance is a function of calories in versus calories out. If you simply take a cheat day without compensating by eating less at other times, you will ultimately gain back unwanted body fat!

Personalizing a Diet to Maintain Your Present Body Composition

What follows is the three-step process for personalizing a diet to maintain your present body composition. For illustrative purposes, we will use the example of a male Type II weighing 175 pounds. Based on DCML, total estimated caloric intake will be 2,625 calories (i.e., $175 \times 15 = 2,625$).

STEP ONE: DETERMINE PROTEIN INTAKE

This number will be fixed regardless of how many calories you consume. Since protein intake corresponds to one gram per pound of goal body weight, total daily protein consumption will amount to 700 calories (i.e., 175 grams $\times$ 4 calories per gram = 700 calories).

STEP TWO: DETERMINE CARBOHYDRATE INTAKE

Type IIs (see Chapter 4) generally do best on a moderate carb diet corresponding to approximately 45 to 50 percent of total calories. Again, we'll start out on the lower end of the spectrum and go with 45 percent. Hence, we multiply total calories by 60 percent and come up with 1,180 calories of carbs (i.e., $.45 \times 2,625$ total calories = 1,180). Since each gram of carbs is four calories, you'll consume approximately 295 grams of carbs.

STEP THREE: DETERMINE FAT INTAKE

Calories from fat are what's left over after total calories from protein and carbs are subtracted from your estimated caloric intake. Since protein amounts to 700 calories and carbs are 1,180 calories, fat will be 640 calories (2,625 total calories minus 1,880 calories from protein and carbs = 745 calories). As each gram of fat is nine calories, approximately 83 grams will come from dietary fat.

Putting it all together, you'd have a diet consisting of 45 percent carbohydrate (295 grams), 27 percent protein (175 grams), and 28 percent fat (83 grams).

The following is a seven-day sample meal plan that illustrates the concepts of a weight-maintenance diet. As in the previous example, caloric intake is estimated at 2,625 calories. Of course, you will need to adjust the amount of calories based on your individual needs.

Day One

MEAL ONE
- 2 cups cream of wheat
- 12 ounces milk (98 percent fat-free)
- 1 or 2 cups coffee or tea

MEAL TWO
- Peach smoothie (1 large peach, 1 scoop whey protein powder, 1 tablespoon flaxseed oil, and crushed ice)

MEAL THREE
- 4 ounces turkey breast
- 8 ounces whole-wheat angel hair pasta
- Large salad (romaine lettuce, green pepper, carrot, tomato, onion, balsamic vinegar, and 1 tablespoon olive oil)

MEAL FOUR
- 8 ounces cheese ravioli
- 2 medium plums

MEAL FIVE
- 8 ounces top round London broil
- 12 ounces green beans

Day Two

MEAL ONE
- Spinach omelet (4 egg whites, 1 whole egg, 4 ounces fresh spinach)
- 1 large bran muffin
- 1 or 2 cups coffee or tea

MEAL TWO
- 1 cup plain yogurt with fresh blueberries
- 1 tablespoon flaxseed oil

MEAL THREE
- Tuna salad (6 ounces tuna, arugula, tomato, and 1 tablespoon olive oil)
- 2 large yams

MEAL FOUR
- 2 cups brown rice
- 1 cup black beans
- 1 large orange

MEAL FIVE
- 12 ounces Chilean sea bass
- 12 ounces broccoli

Day Three

MEAL ONE
- 1½ cups all-bran cereal
- 2 ounces seedless raisins
- 12 ounces milk (98 percent fat-free)
- 1 or 2 cups coffee or tea

MEAL TWO
- Turkey sandwich (6 ounces turkey breast and 2 slices rye bread)
- 1 large apple

MEAL THREE
- 6 ounces shrimp
- 2 cups corn niblets
- Large salad (romaine lettuce, green pepper, carrot, tomato, onion, balsamic vinegar, and 1 tablespoon olive oil)

MEAL FOUR
- Pineapple smoothie (1 cup pineapple, 1 scoop whey protein powder, 1 tablespoon flaxseed oil, and crushed ice)

MEAL FIVE
- 8 ounces Atlantic salmon
- 12 ounces Brussels sprouts

Day Four

MEAL ONE
- 1 cup oatmeal
- 1 scoop whey protein powder
- 1 tablespoon flaxseed oil
- 1 or 2 cups coffee or tea

MEAL TWO
- Turkey chili (4 ounces turkey and 1 cup kidney beans)
- 2 medium apricots

MEAL THREE
- 4-ounce chicken breast
- 8 ounces whole-wheat linguine
- Large salad (containing romaine lettuce, green pepper, carrot, tomato, onion, balsamic vinegar, and 1 tablespoon olive oil)

MEAL FOUR
- 1 cup plain yogurt with sliced fresh strawberries

MEAL FIVE
- 6-ounce filet mignon
- 12 ounces cauliflower

Day Five

MEAL ONE
- 1 large pumpernickel bagel
- 1 cup cottage cheese (98 percent fat-free)
- 1 or 2 cups coffee or tea

MEAL TWO
- 4 ounces turkey breast
- 2 cups brown rice
- 8 ounces fruit salad

MEAL THREE
- Steak sandwich (6-ounce sirloin strip steak on whole-wheat pita)
- Large salad (romaine lettuce, green pepper, carrot, tomato, onion, balsamic vinegar, and 1 tablespoon olive oil)

MEAL FOUR
- Raspberry smoothie (containing 1 cup raspberries, 1 scoop whey protein powder, 1 tablespoon flaxseed oil, and crushed ice)

MEAL FIVE
- 6 ounces catfish
- 12 ounces asparagus

Day Six

MEAL ONE
- Power pancakes (1 cup whole-wheat pancake mix and 1 scoop whey protein powder)
- 1 tablespoon flaxseed oil
- 1 or 2 cups coffee or tea

MEAL TWO
- Soy burger (8-ounce soy patty and 2 slices multigrain bread)
- 1 large apple

MEAL THREE
- Crab salad (containing 4 ounces Alaskan king crab legs, arugula, tomato, and 1 tablespoon olive oil)
- 2 large yams

MEAL FOUR
- 4 ounces flank steak
- 12 ounces green peas
- 1 large pear

MEAL FIVE
- 6 ounces rainbow trout
- 12 ounces zucchini

Day Seven

MEAL ONE
- Mushroom egg white omelet (6 egg whites and 1 portobello mushroom)
- 2 large sweet potatoes
- 1 tablespoon flaxseed oil
- 1 or 2 cups coffee or tea

MEAL TWO
- Buffalo burger (4 ounces ground buffalo meat on 2 slices whole-wheat bread)
- ¼ sliced cantaloupe

MEAL THREE
- Spaghetti with turkey meatballs (8 ounces whole-wheat spaghetti and 4 ounces ground turkey breast)
- Large salad (romaine lettuce, green pepper, carrot, tomato, onion, balsamic vinegar, and 1 tablespoon olive oil)

MEAL FOUR
- 3 ounces mixed nuts (almonds, walnuts, and peanuts)

MEAL FIVE
- 6 ounces halibut
- 12 ounces kale

CHAPTER 9

Nine Ways to a Leaner Body

EAT SMALL, FREQUENT MEALS

In today's fast-paced world, people generally give little thought about the timing of their meals. All too often, breakfast consists of only a cup of coffee. Succeeding meals are eaten whenever there is a free moment, usually culminating with a large feast in the evening and possibly even a midnight snack.

Clearly, such a haphazard approach to nutrition has a detrimental effect on your physique. Ideal body composition can be attained only through dietary regimentation. Simply becoming more regimented with your diet reduces hunger sensations, independent of the types of nutrients consumed.[1] The old-school solution is to organize meals into breakfast, lunch, and dinner. Eating three square meals a day has become a generally accepted nutritional tenet. But to keep your body operating at peak efficiency, you need to push the envelope even further.

Consistent with the set-point theory, your body strives to maintain enough energy (i.e., body fat) to survive the next famine. So when you go without eating for more than a few hours, it senses deprivation and shifts into a "starvation mode." Part of the starvation response is to decrease resting energy expenditure. In effect, the body slows down its metabolic rate to conserve energy.

The starvation response is largely accomplished via hormonal regulation. One of the primary metabolic hormones affected is thyroid hormone, particularly the active form called T3. As previously discussed, T3 helps to mobilize fat stores and increase their use as a fuel source. During the starvation response, the production of thyroid hormone decreases precipitously. As a rule, the longer the period in between meals, the more these effects are heightened.[2]

In addition, meal frequency has a negative effect on insulin levels.[3] Eating a few large meals causes insulin spikes, switching on mechanisms that increase fat storage. But that's not all. During the lengthy between-meal periods associated with eating infrequently, there is a tendency toward hypoglycemia (low blood sugar). In an attempt to restore blood sugar, your body signals the hypothalamus that it needs food, especially simple carbohydrates. Hunger pangs ensue and you invariably end up eating more than you otherwise would, often in the form of refined sweets. This sets up the vicious cycle of overeating and uncontrolled insulin secretions—a surefire route to unwanted weight gain.

Compounding matters, the absence of food causes the stomach to secrete ghrelin. If you remember, ghrelin is a short-term regulator of set point. It exerts its effects by slowing down fat utilization and increasing hunger. Without consistent food consumption, ghrelin levels remain elevated for extended periods of time.

Based on these facts, it's easy to see why frequent feedings are beneficial. They help to stabilize insulin levels and keep appetite under control.[4,5] Blood sugar is well regulated, without any sudden surges or dips. And since there is an almost constant flow of food into the stomach, the hunger-inducing effects of ghrelin are suppressed, reducing the urge to binge.

What's more, a multimeal strategy has a positive impact on metabolism.[6] By constantly taking in food, the body thinks it has a steady source of fuel. Not only does this maintain elevated levels of thyroid hormone, but it also increases postprandial thermogenesis, allowing calories to be expended as heat rather than being stored as fat.[7,8] Although the exact reason for this is unclear, it may at least be partially attributable to the increased energy expenditure associated with digestion (called the thermic effect of food). Every time you eat, your body burns off a portion of the calories, keeping metabolism elevated for up to several hours after consumption. By constantly taking in food, you prolong this thermic effect and thus take maximal advantage of food's metabolic properties.

The importance of frequent feedings is magnified when you're trying to lose weight. The reason: preservation of muscle. During periods of caloric restriction, the body breaks down muscle protein and converts it into glucose for use as an energy source. By increasing meal frequency, you attenuate the rate of muscle tissue breakdown. This allows you to maintain more lean body mass and thereby aid in weight management.[9,10] And here is one instance where more is better; it has been shown that people who consume five meals a day are able to stay leaner than those who consume only three.[11]

Eating frequently also has valuable health-related implications. Specifically, it produces a significant decrease in LDL cholesterol (the "bad" cholesterol) while raising the ever-so-important HDL/LDL cholesterol ratio.[12,13] This lipid-lowering effect has been shown to reduce atherosclerotic plaques, a fact that directly decreases cardiovascular risk.[14]

The best way to implement frequent feedings into your regimen is by spacing out meals evenly, eating five or six times a day at regular intervals. Consuming a meal every two or three hours or so is ideal. While this might seem like a chore, it actually can be accomplished rather easily. A "meal" doesn't need to be gourmet; it can be as simple as a yogurt or a piece of fruit. As long as you're choosing "quality" food sources, you'll derive benefits.

A good strategy is to prepare several meals in advance, store them in plastic containers, and reheat them in a microwave oven in a glass dish on an as-needed basis. This allows you to consolidate preparation, thereby heightening efficiency.

Another alternative is to supplement your basic meals with powdered meal replacements (MRPs). These "engineered foods" provide the ultimate in convenience: they are nutritionally balanced, easily transportable, and can be prepared in a matter of minutes. Over the long term, these factors make them an excellent aid in the pursuit of lasting weight management. In fact, fat-loss programs that use MRPs are significantly more successful than those that don't.[15,16]

A third option is to opt for one of the numerous nutritional bars on the market. These bars come in a wide array of different flavors and, with advances in technol-

Helpful Hint

Don't be concerned if, at the onset, you find it difficult to eat so frequently. It has been postulated that any activity done consistently for one month becomes habit and diet is no exception. For some it might take a little longer and for others not quite so long, but if you adhere to the same nutritional protocol on a consistent basis, it will become ingrained into your subconscious. Eventually, eating every few hours will be second nature.

ogy, are often quite tasty. However, be careful which one you choose. Many products are nothing more than glorified candy bars, containing ample amounts of sugar and saturated fat. Make sure to check labels before you buy. As previously discussed, stay away from anything that lists high fructose corn syrup and/or partially hydrogenated oil as one of the first ingredients.

REDUCE STARCHES AT NIGHT

For many Americans, starchy carbs make up a substantial portion of their evening meals. Pasta, rice, potatoes . . . these are nightly staples in the standard Western diet. Steak and fries, spaghetti and meatballs—what would dinner be without them?

The trouble with starchy carbs is that they are more readily transformed to fat when eaten before bedtime. The reason for this is simple: The primary function of carbohydrates is to supply short-term energy for your daily activities. If carbs are not used immediately for fuel, they have two possible fates: They either are stored as glycogen in your liver and muscles or are indirectly (or in some cases directly) converted into fatty acids and stored in adipose tissue as body fat.[17] Since activity levels usually are lowest during the evening hours, there is a diminished use of carbs for fuel. Hypothetically, this sets up an environment in which the body is more inclined to convert carbs into fat.

Compounding matters is the diurnal nature of insulin sensitivity. For reasons that aren't entirely clear, insulin sensitivity is highest in the morning.[18,19] This means your body is better able to assimilate carbs at this time, thereby keeping blood sugar levels stable. As the day wears on, insulin sensitivity gradually diminishes and, by evening, it's at its lowest point. Hence, carbs eaten at night evoke a greater insulin response, fueling the processes that facilitate fat storage and suppress fat burning.

What's more, consuming starches at night has a carry-over effect to the next day. Eating a carbohydrate-rich dinner tends to increase the insulin response of the following morning's meal.[20] So not only are insulin levels elevated after dinner, but they remain that way through breakfast, too.

Another factor to consider is the effect of carbohydrate on appetite. While protein (and, to a certain degree, fat) help to suppress hunger, carbs tend to increase it.[21] Through various mechanisms, the breakdown of starches into glucose enhances the urge to eat. This increases the potential to have a late-night snack—one of the biggest culprits in unwanted weight gain.

In general, it's best to consume carbs early in the day, when your activity levels and insulin sensitivity are at their peak. Breakfast is the time to load up on nutrient-dense carbs. After an overnight fast, glycogen is depleted from your liver (and, to a lesser extent, your muscles). Since glycogen has important physiologic significance to the onset of starvation, the body strives to replenish these glycogen stores and tends to utilize carbs for this purpose rather than for fat storage after you have "broken the fast." A large bowl of rolled oats or bran cereal with some fruit is ideal. It'll help to fuel your daily activities and keep you physically and mentally fit throughout the day.

On the other hand, it is best to limit your dinner fare to fibrous, vegetable-based food sources (this isn't applicable for those seeking to bulk up). Fibrous vegetables tend to be extremely low in total calories and, because of their bulk, are very filling. For supper, consider eating a meal consisting of lean poultry or fish combined with a large bowl of salad greens. Other vegetables (e.g., broccoli, string beans, cauliflower, zucchini) also make fine nighttime carbohydrate choices, and will reduce the potential for unwanted body-fat storage.

COOK RIGHT

The way you cook can have a major impact on both your health and body composition. Let's review some of the most popular methods of cooking and discuss how they can be implemented for optimal results.

Grilling/Broiling

Grilling can be a healthy and delicious way to cook foods. Meats and vegetables, in particular, are great on the grill. But there is a potential downside: grilling meats can result in the production of dangerous compounds called heterocyclic amines (HCAs). HCAs are carcinogenic and have been linked to cancers of the breast, colon, bladder, prostate, and pancreas.[22]

The formation of cancer-causing agents is increased if grilling is done over an open flame. When fat from the meat drips down and hits the coals (even lean meats contain some fat), it releases compounds called polycyclic aromatic hydrocarbons (PAHs), which are just as bad for your health as HCAs. As a rule, the longer food stays on the grill and the higher the cooking temperature, the greater the amount of PAHs and HCAs that are formed.

Here are several strategies that can be implemented for healthier grilling.

- *Marinate your meats:* In addition to enhancing flavor, marinating meat forms a protective barrier that reduces HCAs by as much as 99 percent.[23] A combination of garlic, herbs, vinegar, and/or citrus fruits can make for an excellent marinade. Avoid using oily marinades and thick commercial sauces, though, as they can drip down and cause PAH-induced flare-ups.

- *Preheat in the microwave:* Microwaving meats for one or two minutes prior to grilling reduces cooking time—a major factor in HCA production. This simple practice has been shown to produce up to a ninefold decrease in potential carcinogens.[24]

- *Turn down the heat:* Grilling foods at lower temperatures can drastically cut HCA formation while still killing off unhealthy bacteria such as *E. coli* and *Salmonella*.[25] Decreasing cooking temperature to around 320 degrees Fahrenheit has been shown to be a safe and effective way to prepare meats with little or no increase in cooking time.

- *Turn meats frequently:* Flipping meats several times significantly reduces HCAs. Just make sure to use tongs or a spatula instead of a fork. This prevents the meat from being pierced, which can allow juices to seep into the flames.

- *Remove any charred material:* When you overcook a meat, HCAs burn into its surface. Fortunately, all you have to do is scrape off the charred substances and you'll get rid of these cancer-causing agents.

Frying

Despite what many think, frying can be an acceptable way to cook—provided it's done right. Most people, however, don't follow proper protocols—a surefire recipe for nutritional disaster.

One of the most important aspects of frying is to choose the right oil. For this, you need to be familiar with a concept called smoke point. An oil's smoke point is the heating stage where it begins to emit smoke and unpleasant odors.

As a rule, oils containing polyunsaturated fatty acids (PUFAs) have the lowest smoke point. Excessive heat breaks the delicate double-bond structure of these fats, turning them rancid.[26] Vitamins and minerals literally go up in smoke. So do antioxidants (especially vitamin E and carotenoids). Toxic carcinogens are formed that wreak havoc on your cells. In short, all the benefits of these healthy fats are lost. Accordingly, flaxseed, sunflower, sesame, peanut, and other high PUFA oils should never be used in frying

Oils that are predominantly monounsaturated have higher smoke points. Olive and canola oils, in particular, tend to hold up relatively well under low levels of heat and therefore are viable for sautéing or stir-frying foods.[27] An even better option is to use a nonstick cooking spray that contains one of these oils. These products allow you to apply a fine layer of oil to the pan—enough to prevent sticking without adding many calories to the meal.

Refrain from frying at high levels of heat. As with grilling, this practice results in the formation of HCAs and PAHs.[28] If, for some reason, you absolutely must do so, the best oil to use is grape seed extract. It has the highest smoke point of all fats and is stable up to temperatures of about 485 degrees Fahrenheit.

No matter what, avoid deep-fat frying. From both a caloric as well as health perspective, this is absolutely the worst way to cook. What's more, stay away from fried foods from fast-food restaurants at all costs. These establishments fry under high heat and use oils containing more than 30 percent of dangerous trans fats.[29] And in an effort to save money, they'll routinely reuse the oil over and over again, thereby producing toxic compounds that have a host of deleterious effects on your body.[30]

Baking/Roasting

Baking involves cooking foods in an oven with dry heat. Roasting is similar to baking but, because it is done at higher temperatures, decreases cook time. Both of these techniques are viable ways to prepare various foods. For best results, cover the dish with tinfoil or a fitted top. This helps to keep the juices in foods, leaving them moist and tender.

If possible, place foods in nonstick cookware such as Teflon. This way, you won't have to use an oil or shortening during cooking, minimizing the amount of calories in the meal. Don't worry about the coating seeping into the food as it is nontoxic and passes through your body without being absorbed.

Steaming

Steaming is a terrific option for cooking many of your favorite foods. It is efficient and clean, allowing you to cook without using any oil. And since foods are not immersed in water, it results in virtually no loss of nutrients.

Steaming can be done in a variety of implements but a metal or bamboo steaming basket generally works best. Use as large a pot as possible to allow adequate room for the steam to circulate. Otherwise, the food won't cook evenly.

Microwaving

In this day and age, it's almost incomprehensible to imagine life without a microwave oven. It is the ultimate in speed and convenience, letting you quickly and easily heat up a meal.

Because it pulls water out of foods, microwaving isn't recommended for meats as it leaves them dry and tough. Almost anything else tastes great when nuked, though. From veggies to hot cereal to canned goods, the microwave oven is a godsend for those times when you need to cook with minimal hassle.

A word of caution: When microwaving, don't use any type of plastics. There is evidence that chemicals in these products (called plasticizers) migrate into the food source, with potentially toxic consequences.[31] Even plastic products that claim to be "microwave safe" have been found to be unsafe. Instead, microwave your foods in glass or ceramic containers.

Boiling

Generally speaking, boiling isn't an ideal way to cook, because it can result in the considerable loss of nutrients. Water-soluble vitamins, in particular, are readily absorbed into boiled water. And unless you drink the water that the food was boiled in, you end up missing out on these valuable nutrients.

The best advice is to limit boiling to grains (such as pasta, rice, and hot cereals). As opposed to other food sources, grains maintain most of their nutritional value when boiled. Just make sure to prepare them al dente. The longer you boil a starch, the more you raise its glycemic rating. For instance, rice boiled for one minute takes twice the time to digest as rice boiled for six minutes. This not only diminishes satiety, but it also raises insulin levels—factors that can ultimately translate into increased fat storage.

If you want to cook a food in water, consider poaching it. Since the liquid that you poach in is eaten as part of the dish, all the nutrients are preserved. To minimize time of preparation, use as little water as possible.

GO EASY ON THE SAUCE

The world floats on a sea of alcohol. Whether it's the two-martini lunch, the evening happy hour, or the after-dinner drink, alcohol is firmly ingrained in today's society. It is, without question, the most popular recreational drug in existence. In many circles, getting drunk even is a rite of passage—a rite that often continues throughout adulthood. With such widespread social acceptance, it's no wonder that approximately half of all Americans drink on a regular basis and more than 5 percent are considered heavy drinkers.

However, for anyone aspiring to maximize his or her body's potential, alcohol is a definite taboo. Make no mistake; alcohol will make you fat. It is calorically dense, containing more than seven calories per gram (as opposed to carbs and protein, which have four). And this doesn't include the addition of mixers, which can significantly increase the calorie count. Take a look at the caloric content in some popular alcoholic beverages: a margarita has 600 calories, a martini 250, and a beer 150—pretty heavy stuff! What's more, these drinks are virtually devoid of any nutritional value. They are "empty calories" that do nothing but pack on unwanted pounds. Considering these facts, there is no doubt that even moderate drinking can have a decidedly negative impact on your figure.

In addition, alcohol tends to promote excessive food intake.[32,33] It is associated with longer meal durations and unregulated eating.[34] Thus, rather than displacing calories from whole foods, alcohol supplements them.

Moreover, since the body has a difficult time breaking down alcohol, it tends to impede fat burning. The liver must use a tremendous amount of coenzymes (especially NAD+) in order to assimilate the alcohol-related toxins. Consequently, there are fewer of these coenzymes available to carry out vital metabolic functions, including the breakdown of fat for energy. The end result: increased fat storage.[35,36] This process can begin after just a single night of heavy drinking.

With chronic abuse, the consequences of alcohol can be disastrous—often irreparable. Alcohol is a poison. It infiltrates your internal organs and has a toxic effect on everything that it comes into contact with. Your liver and spleen, in particular, become severely impaired and lose their ability to carry out vital functions. Forget about losing body fat; your entire metabolic system becomes dysfunctional. And don't think your muscles are immune from the carnage. Alcohol consumption significantly decreases testosterone production and muscle-protein synthesis—the primary mechanisms in muscular development.[37,38,39] And sustained bouts of heavy drinking can even lead to rhabdomyolysis—a serious disorder that damages the structural integrity of muscle tissue.[40]

On the other hand, there is evidence that moderate alcohol intake can be healthy for your heart. Initially, it was thought that these benefits were limited to red wine, which contains polyphenolic compounds (such as resveratrol and proanthocyanidins) that function as antioxidants and act to reduce the formation of artery-clogging plaques.[41] Additional research, however, has shown that beer, whiskey, and other liquors provide cardioprotection, as well.[42] Apparently, alcohol helps to thin the blood, thereby reducing the potential for clotting. So regardless of the type of drink, consuming alcoholic beverages can mitigate the risk of cardiovascular disease.

All things considered, the best advice on alcohol is to limit consumption to no more than a few drinks a week. Any heart-healthy benefits are counterbalanced by its addictive properties and negative impact on body composition. Get used to the idea that you don't need alcohol to have a good time. If you're out at a party or dance club, order a club soda with a twist of lemon or lime. This way, you'll be in full control of your faculties when others are in a drunken stupor. You'll wake up hangover-free, never having to regret what you did the night before. And, of course, you'll keep your body operating at peak efficiency, maintaining a terrific physique year-round.

JUMP-START WITH JAVA

For years, health-care practitioners have denounced caffeine as a health hazard. They've cautioned against its use, citing studies that link it to everything from heart disease to cancer. In some circles, caffeine is even lumped together with alcohol and nicotine as the "dangerous triad." Eliminate caffeine from your daily life and you'll be happier and healthier—or so the thinking goes.

The truth is, however, caffeine has gotten a bad rap. Despite the negative press, the anti-caffeine sentiment is largely unfounded. A close examination of research reveals that any carcinogenic effects of caffeine are vastly overstated. Some of the studies showing a positive correlation between caffeine and cancer were plagued with errors in statistical analysis.[43] Others gave rats enormous quantities of caffeine—far beyond what the normal individual consumes. Sure, if you drink fifty cups of coffee a day it's going to have a deleterious effect on your health. But this means little in practical terms. When all the available information is examined, there's really no evidence that modest caffeine consumption causes any detriments to overall well-being.[44] A few studies actually found a negative correlation between caffeine and certain forms of cancer![45]

Does this mean that you should load up on caffeinated beverages? Absolutely not! Caffeine is a stimulant. At high doses, it can cause a host of unwanted side effects, such as hypertension, nervousness, insomnia, and gastrointestinal distress.[46] Guzzling mass quantities of coffee and cola will only serve to make you wired and irritable—not lean and defined.

However, when used in moderation, caffeine can be a safe and effective means of expediting a loss of body fat. It exerts its effects by acting on the sympathetic nervous system to increase catecholamine (i.e., epinephrine and norepinephrine) production.[47] Catecholamines facilitate the release of free fatty acids from adipocytes, allowing fat to be utilized for short-term energy. And this metabolic thrust isn't transient; it lasts up to several hours after ingestion.[48]

You don't need to take a lot of caffeine to derive positive benefits. A daily dose of 200 to 300 milligrams is all that's required to rev up your metabolic rate.[49] Two cups of brewed coffee first thing in the morning or before your workout will satisfy this requirement quite nicely. For best results, black coffee or espresso is recommended; adding cream or sugar will easily offset the caffeine-induced increase in metabolic rate. If black coffee is simply too bitter for your taste buds, then try using skim milk and artificial sweeteners as flavor enhancers.

An even better alternative to coffee is herbal green tea. In addition to having a good amount of caffeine, green tea also contains compounds called catechins that serve to further increase metabolism. Catechins inhibit an enzyme (called catechol-O-methyl-transferase) that is responsible for degrading noradrenaline, a potent hormone that promotes the oxidation of body fat.[50] In combination, caffeine and catechins act synergistically to enhance resting energy expenditure beyond what is achieved by caffeine alone.[51] Considering that it also is replete in vitamins and antioxidants, green tea is a terrific beverage for keeping your body in peak condition. There is even evidence that, because of its concentration of flavonoids, it helps to increase bone density and stave off cardiovascular disease![52,53]

It's generally best to abstain from using a caffeinated product several hours before bedtime. Because of its stimulatory effects, it can interfere with your circadian rhythms and throw your sleep/wake cycle out of whack. This leads to desynchronization of your biorhythms, a condition where sleep is less restful at night and mental acuity is compromised during the day.

Table 9.1 shows some of the most popular sugar-free sources of caffeine.

Table 9.1

SUGAR-FREE SOURCES OF CAFFEINE	
SOURCE	**AMOUNT OF CAFFEINE** (Milligrams)
Brewed coffee (8 ounces)	135
Tea (8 ounces)	55
Snapple Diet Iced Tea	48
Diet Coke (12 ounces)	47
Pepsi Light	36

CHEW YOUR FOOD!

As opposed to the leisurely meals consumed by Europeans, American meals are often eaten in a hurry. We tend to scoff down food as quickly as possible, without chewing fully. But the act of chewing, or mastication, is important on several levels.

First, chewing improves digestion. As you chew, food is broken down into smaller and smaller pieces. This is accompanied by an increased production of saliva, which has enzymes (e.g., salivary amylase) that accelerate the breakdown of carbohydrate and fat.[54] The combination of these factors reduces the load on the gut, thereby ensuring better nutrient assimilation.

By prolonging the time needed to eat a meal, chewing also increases satiety.[55,56,57] As previously discussed, there are various mechanisms by which the consumption of food transmits satiety signals to the brain (including the secretion of hormones and the activation of stretch receptors). But these mechanisms aren't instantaneous. Rather, it takes a little time before they exert their full effects. Hence, if you eat too fast, by the time your stomach is sated, you've probably already eaten too much. This is one of the primary reasons why juices are not recommended for weight loss; calories are taken in so quickly that satiety mechanisms are bypassed, thereby encouraging the potential to overeat.[58]

So try to take your time when eating. Cut your food into small pieces and aim to chew each bite about ten to fifteen times. Do this on a regular basis and your meals will be more satisfying—both from a satiety and enjoyment standpoint.

SPICE IT UP

Using spices in your dishes is one of the best ways to improve their taste. But spices are more than just flavor enhancers. In fact, using the right ones can actually have a positive impact on your physique. For example, acidic compounds such as vinegar and lemon juice slow gastric emptying, allowing food to remain in the gut for longer periods of time. In addition to promoting satiety, this also improves the glycemic response of a meal.[59] And a lower glycemic response translates to stable insulin levels, reducing the potential for fat deposition.

Capsaicin, the pungent ingredient in red pepper, has been shown to aid in weight loss in two distinct ways. First, it has thermogenic properties, increasing your body's ability to burn fat.[60,61] In addition, capsaicin helps to curb appetite, reducing the amounts of food consumed throughout the day.[62]

Ginger is another spice that has proven to be thermogenic.[63] It contains extracts called gingerols that stimulate fat burning and aid in digestion. And as an added benefit, it is rich in vitamins and minerals, including various antioxidants that promote cellular health.

The bottom line is that you should be liberal with the inclusion of spices in your meals. Not only will they enhance the flavor of foods, but you may improve your body composition in the process, as well. So go ahead and be generous with the hot sauce; sprinkle on the balsamic; garnish with ginger—your taste buds, as well as your physique, will reap the rewards.

SET GOALS

When starting a diet, people are usually brimming with enthusiasm. They're eager to see results and committed to doing whatever it takes to stay on the right nutritional track. During this honeymoon period, everything is destined to go very well.

Within a short time, however, the novelty starts to wear off. Personal issues, impatience, and a host of other factors contribute to a diminished zeal. And as enthusiasm wanes, so does dietary adherence. Little by little, eating habits return to previous norms. Eventually, dieting goes completely by the wayside and so does any hope of getting into optimal shape.

One of the best ways to keep up your motivation to eat healthfully is by setting goals.[64,65] If you have clearly defined goals, you are much more likely to stay on the nutritional straight and narrow. Even if outside factors cause you to temporarily stray from your diet, the allure of achieving your goals is apt to get you back on track.

For the strategy to work properly, goals must be both quantifiable and attainable. Goals that do not meet both of these conditions are nonspecific and therefore not meaningful. It's difficult to achieve nonspecific goals, and failure is apt to result in frustration. Let's discuss the qualities of a specific goal in detail:

- For a goal to be quantifiable, it must have measurable parameters. For example, losing 20 pounds in three months is a quantifiable goal. You can weigh yourself today and again in three months to see whether you have met your goal. The scale will indicate your weight loss in a measurable context. Other examples of quantifiable goals include reducing your waistline by two inches in a month or dropping one dress size in six weeks. Conversely, wanting to look good is not a quantifiable goal. This is subjective and not measurable by any defined standards. A "goal" like this is doomed to lead to disappointment and frustration.

- For a goal to be attainable, it must be realistic. For example, losing 20 pounds in three months is an attainable goal; losing 90 pounds in three months is not. If a goal is not attainable, it can serve as a de-motivator and cause you to feel that your efforts are pointless. To avoid this fate, it's better to set modest goals that are readily within reach. Attaining them produces a feeling of accomplishment and spurs you on to loftier goals. Furthermore, long-term goals should be broken down into shorter-term ones. Losing 60 pounds in a year might seem like a cumbersome task but losing 5 pounds in one month doesn't. Again, the prospect of attainability will keep you focused.

Several techniques are useful in reinforcing your goals and thus sustaining dietary adherence. One such method is visualization. Visualize your entire body—your arms, legs, shoulders, and so on—and get an image of the way you want them to appear. Think of yourself in great shape, walking on the beach in a bikini or wearing a sexy dress at a party. You might want to think of someone whose physique you admire (preferably someone with a similar body type) and envision yourself developing a comparable physique. Let your imagination be your internal source of motivation and, within reason, do not set any limits to what you can accomplish.

If you find it difficult to use your imagination as a motivator, find a picture of yourself when you were happy with the way you looked and tape it to the refrigerator or put in on your dresser. It is common to feel as if you are fighting an uphill battle and lose perspective about your ability to succeed. By having a tangible image in full view, you'll reinforce the idea that you have the potential to look terrific. Every time you see this picture, it will remind you of your potential. And I can assure you that if you follow my nutritional program, you will soon look your best.

In short, think about what motivates you and commit these things to your memory. Every time you feel the urge to stray from your diet, remember your goals. Then consider the following: Is the temporary satisfaction of having a brief taste sensation, whatever it may be, worth the consequences to your physique and health? If your goals are meaningful, the answer will be a resounding "No!" You'll be able to forgo the temptation of short-term pleasure for the myriad long-term rewards that are sure to ensue from following the LGN Diet.

Remember, though, you have to really yearn for something to maintain enthusiasm over time. Without a specific goal, you won't have sufficient impetus to put in the sacrifice necessary to achieve results. Give yourself an edge and make use of every possible motivator that is meaningful to you—it will inspire you to eat healthy for life.

Once you accomplish a goal, you should immediately set new goals. This will keep you focused in your efforts and allow you to maintain a zest for eating right. You should also review your goals periodically to make sure they are consistent with your present objectives. Your goals will often change over time, and by consistently reevaluating your position, you'll be much more likely to remain on course.

WRITE IT DOWN

Whenever I counsel a new client on nutrition, the first thing I do is ask him or her to fill out a food diary. The usual reaction is "Aw, come on. I know what I eat. Why do I need to fill out a food diary?"

The truth is, however, most people are completely unaware of their own eating habits. They almost always underestimate the quantity of food consumed and are oblivious to the types and ratios of macronutrients they eat. In a way, this is understandable. Eating is generally done on impulse. It's an unconscious, conditioned activity that encompasses a wide range of both psychological and physiological factors.[66] See food, eat food—this is an innate human trait.

Here is where the value of a food diary comes in. It forces you to be aware of everything you put into your mouth. This way, impulsive eating behavior is transformed into a conscious mode. And seeing what you eat in black and white can be quite a revelation. The diary doesn't lie (assuming you're honest in what you write down!), providing a complete snapshot of your dietary habits, from soup to nuts, so to speak.

When designing a food diary, it's best to follow the follow the KIS principle: keep it simple (see sample food diary below). You don't need extraneous data. Here are the five essential components that should be included:

- *Day:* Write down the day of the week that you are reporting (Monday, Tuesday, Wednesday, etc.).
- *Time:* Write down both the time you started eating each meal as well as the time you finished eating.
- *Place:* Write down where you ate each meal. Was it at home, in a restaurant, at work, during transport?
- *Description:* Write down a description of the foods that you ate. Include as much information as possible, such as the way the food was prepared (e.g., raw, broiled, fried, etc.), the cut of meat, the type of bread, and so

on. Don't forget to include any condiments, sauces, or gravies. Salad dressing, mayonnaise, ketchup, soy sauce, butter, and sour cream all can add a significant amount of calories to a meal and must be accounted for.

- *Quantity:* Write down the amount of each food consumed. This is the most important factor in weight management so try to be specific here. If you are weighing your foods (as you should at the onset of your diet), then write down how many ounces, tablespoons, etc. Alternatively, if you are eyeballing it, use estimates such as "large piece of steak," "handful of nuts," and so forth. The more descriptive you can be, the better.

FOOD DIARY				
Day	Time	Place	Food Description	Quantity

Contrary to what you may think, using a food diary doesn't require a lot of time or effort; a few minutes is all that's required to fill in the necessary info. You can write everything down before, during, or after each meal; it's your choice. Just don't wait until the end of the day to do it as relying on your memory is a recipe for disaster. You'll inevitably forget important data, compromising the accuracy of the information.

Once a week, review your diary in an unbiased fashion. How did you do? If you adhered to your personalized nutritional program the majority of the time, great! You're well on your way to looking great naked. On the other hand, if you deviated significantly from the plan, then further scrutiny is in order. What are the discrepancies between what you're doing and what you should be doing? Go through each meal to gain insight into what caused you to go astray. Look at what triggered eating. Was it your mood? The availability of food? The company you kept? Here are some things to consider:

- *Check the timing of your meals:* This provides vital information about whether you skip meals or don't eat frequently enough. Remember, it is best to consume multiple small meals throughout the day. Regimentation is essential to keep insulin in check, suppress hunger, and stoke your metabolism.
- *See where you ate:* Location can tell a lot about your food choices. Eating out frequently, scoffing down food in your car, dining with friends, snacking in front of the TV, and other settings all can have potential ramifications on diet. Dealing properly with these situations is of prime importance in achieving your nutritional goals.
- *Assess your quantities:* This is generally the place where most people go astray. If you aren't weighing your foods, it is quite possible that you're underestimating how much you're eating. Get a firm handle on the amount of food you're consuming and positive results are sure to follow.

I suggest keeping the diary at least throughout the first several weeks of initiating your diet. Doing so will foster better eating habits and help to make you conscious of food intake for life.

CHAPTER 10

Eat Right to Exercise

Exercise and nutrition go hand in hand: While exercise has a major effect on your body composition, nutrition has a major impact on your exercise performance. Thus, one feeds off the other (no pun intended!).

Make no mistake: If you want to look great naked and maintain optimal health, exercise isn't just beneficial—it's absolutely essential. This can be explained, in part, by the laws of thermodynamics. Remember that there are two sides of the weight-loss equation: energy intake and energy expenditure. By increasing the expenditure part of the equation, exercise helps to create a negative caloric balance and to shift the body into fat-burning mode.

Exercise also helps to improve circulation. Why is this important? Well, in order for body fat to be metabolized, it must first enter the bloodstream and then be transported to the liver and other active tissues for use as fuel. Unfortunately, blood flow tends to be poor in fatty areas, thereby inhibiting your body's ability to harness fat from these regions.

Enter the magic of exercise. It helps to expand your network of capillaries—the tiny blood vessels that allow nutrients to be exchanged between bodily tissues. The more capillaries you have, the more efficient your body becomes in liberating and utilizing fat, particularly from stubborn areas such as the thighs and love handles.

In addition, consistent exercise expands the size and number of your mitochondria (cellular furnaces where fat burning takes place), and increases the quantity of your aerobic enzymes (bodily proteins that accelerate the fat-burning process). Over time, these factors ratchet up your body's fat-burning ability while improving muscular endurance and function.

Cardio is the most common type of exercise prescribed for losing weight. Depending on your training intensity, a single half-hour session on the treadmill, stair climber, or any other aerobic modality can burn more than 20 grams of fat—enough to offset the amount in a greasy burger and fries. Do this several times a week and you'll certainly expedite fat loss.

But while there's no disputing the fat-burning benefits of cardiovascular exercise, lifting weights can have an even greater impact. This is partly due to a phenomenon called excess postexercise oxygen consumption (EPOC). In a nutshell, EPOC acts to keep your metabolism elevated *after* a workout. Here's the catch, though: EPOC is intensity dependent—the harder you train, the more calories you expend following training. And, since weight training is much more intense than aerobics, it promotes a significantly greater EPOC.[1] Better yet, the duration of EPOC is much longer for weight training, with effects lasting for more than thirty-eight hours![2] So even though you might not expend as much energy during exercise performance, weight training ultimately allows you to burn a greater amount of fat in total.

EXERCISE AND SET POINT

Exercise isn't just a short-term fix to lose body fat; it also helps you stay lean over time. In fact, it can actually help to lower your set point. Let's discuss the myriad ways in which this is accomplished:

Improved Leptin Sensitivity

As previously discussed, leptin has a saturation level above which its uptake into the brain doesn't increase. Once this level is reached, leptin is effectively rendered useless; no matter how much additional leptin you produce, your body will continue to store more fat. Unfortunately, a large percentage of the population has at least some degree of leptin resistance.

The good news is that exercise actually helps to improve your sensitivity to leptin—a fact that has a profound effect on set point.[3,4] When more leptin gets to the brain, less is needed to keep appetite under control. This is why habitual exercisers are better able to regulate their eating habits, even when allowed unlimited access to food.[5]

Reduced Stress

Believe it or not, stress can make you fat! That's right, the pressures of everyday life can contribute to unwanted weight gain and even result in a higher set point. Here's why: When you are under a lot of stress, your body secretes a hormone called cortisol. Among its many functions, cortisol is responsible for cannibalizing muscle tissue for fuel. This, in itself, can lead to a suppression of metabolic rate and therefore increased fat storage. But that's not the worst of it.

Ever notice that when you're stressed out you tend to eat more food? Well, this isn't just a psychological phenomenon. Cortisol acts on your hunger mechanisms. It promotes the release of the appetite-stimulating hormone neuropeptide Y (NPY), while inhibiting satiety hormones such as the melanocortins.[6] In addition, it increases the activity of the fat-storing enzyme lipoprotein lipase. Hence, the extra nutrients you're bound to take in are directed toward fat deposition rather than energy use.[7] And, on top of everything, it impairs the functionality of leptin, throwing your lipostat out of whack.[8,9] The upshot is an increase in body fat and, quite possibly, set point.

Compounding matters, the accumulation of fat from excess cortisol tends to be localized to the abdominal region.[10] This has far-reaching complications, not only on your appearance, but also on your health. If you remember, central obesity has been associated with an increased risk of cardiovascular mortality. Simply stated, a big gut predisposes you to a heart attack.

Exercise works wonders in this regard, helping to counteract stress and reduce excessive cortisol production.[11] Its mode of action is due, at least in part, to the secretion of beta-endorphins—a group of opiatelike compounds that help to promote pleasure and reduce pain. Endorphins are extremely powerful, having more than 100 times the potency of morphine. During a workout, these chemicals are released from the pituitary gland and into the bloodstream, where they attach to brain "receptors" and generate a feeling of euphoria often referred to as an "exercise high."[12] This is one of the reasons that exercise becomes addicting after a while; you simply feel better about yourself after training.

Weight training is particularly effective as a "destressor." As you lift, your mind must be focused to do nothing but perform the task at hand. Worries about work, family, and everything else, for that matter, become secondary. There's simply no opportunity to dwell on negative thoughts during training and any feelings of pent-up frustration, anger, and hostility are channeled into the weights.

Enhanced Glucose Tolerance

Your body's ability to utilize blood glucose has a significant effect on fat storage. If you remember, carbohydrates (and, to a lesser extent, protein and fats) are broken down into simple sugars after consumption. Insulin is then released from your pancreas to remove these sugars from the blood and assist in their storage as glycogen in muscle and liver. This is where it gets a little complicated . . .

To facilitate glucose uptake, muscle cells contain transporter proteins called GLUT4. Think of GLUT4 as little glucose ferries: They rise to the surface of cells to meet sugar molecules and then shuttle them to the inside of the cells for storage as glycogen. Under certain circumstances, however, cells lose some of their capacity to take in glucose. This condition, called insulin resistance, is thought to be a precursor to *Syndrome X*—a group of metabolic afflictions (including increased cholesterol, elevated blood pressure, and increased abdominal fat deposition) that have been implicated in a host of cardiovascular anomalies.

With insulin resistance, your muscles are not able to effectively store glucose as glycogen. Consequently, sugar just keeps circulating in the bloodstream with only one possible fate: storage as body fat. This creates a vicious cycle of increased fat deposition and elevated insulin levels that ultimately leads to a raised set point.

Contrary to popular belief, the primary cause of insulin resistance isn't due to an inability of insulin to bind to target cells. Rather, it is caused by a breakdown in GLUT4 function. In effect, there is a "short circuit" in the insulin signal that normally causes GLUT4 to rise to the cell surface. Without the assistance of GLUT4, glucose simply cannot enter into muscle cells.

By increasing the activity of GLUT4, exercise counteracts insulin resistance.[13] As you work out, muscular contractions "wake up" these transporters, allowing your muscles to take in glucose at an accelerated rate—up to five times more than under resting conditions. And although the full-blown effects are somewhat transient, increased glucose utilization can last for up to forty-eight hours after a workout.

Increased Resting Metabolic Rate

Throughout this book, I've emphasized the importance of muscle in long-term weight management. It is, by far, the most metabolically active tissue in your body.[14] For each pound of muscle, you burn up to an additional 50 calories a day. Better yet, you burn these calories on a continual basis, even when you're lying on the couch watching your favorite TV program! To put this in perspective, by gaining a mere 5 pounds of lean muscle (which, if you're a beginner, can be accomplished in a matter of months), you'll burn an additional 1,750 calories a week. Assuming you keep food consumption constant, those 5 pounds of muscle will result in a net loss of about 25 pounds of fat in just one year's time!

The metabolic properties of muscle are integrally tied to your set point. A loss of muscle causes your set point to drift higher. This inevitably leads to a weight-loss plateau and makes it more difficult to lose weight in the future. Conversely, increasing your muscle mass effectively lowers your set point, thereby making it easier to lose body fat and keep it off over the long haul. I've had clients tell me they couldn't get below a certain level of body fat and, voilà, after adding some muscle, the pounds seemed to melt away.

It's important to realize that only certain types of exercise are beneficial in this regard. Aerobics, while fine for helping to create a caloric deficit, does virtually nothing to preserve muscle mass. In fact, performing cardio can actually accelerate the loss of muscle if calories are reduced below baseline.[15] Nope, aerobics aren't the answer here; to prevent diet-induced muscle catabolism, you must lift weights.[16,17,18] As a testament to this fact, consider that many bodybuilders never do any form of aerobic exercise yet they remain extremely lean year-round. Their extensive muscularity provides such a great metabolic effect that aerobics simply aren't necessary.

WHAT TO EAT
BEFORE A WORKOUT

The main nutritional goal pre-workout is to supply adequate energy for your muscles and brain during training. This makes carbohydrate consumption essential. If you remember, carbs are stored as glycogen in your liver and muscles. Since high-intensity exercise utilizes energy at a very fast rate, the body can't supply enough oxygen to harness fat as a fuel source. Thus, it relies on its glycogen stores, which don't require oxygen to be broken down for energy.

By taking in an ample amount of carbs before exercise, you ensure that your body's glycogen stores are fully stocked. With a ready supply of glycogen, your muscles can access energy on demand. In this way, you're able to go all out in your training efforts, extending performance without "hitting the wall."

Protein should also be included in your pre-workout meal. Although it doesn't contribute much in the way of energy, consuming protein prior to exercise has both anabolic and anticatabolic effects. By providing a steady stream of amino acids at the onset of training, you maximize their delivery to working muscles and thereby attenuate the breakdown of muscle tissue during your workout. Moreover, you significantly increase muscle-protein synthesis in the first hour *after* exercise, priming the body for anabolism.[19]

The consumption of fat, on the other hand, should be kept to a minimum at this time. Fat delays gastric emptying, thereby prolonging the time it takes foods to digest. If food sits in your stomach during exercise, there is an increased likelihood of gastric problems, including cramping, nausea, and reflux.

Now let's talk specifics. The composition of your pre-workout meal should contain a nutrient-dense starch and a low-fat protein source. Turkey on multigrain bread, lean steak and yams, egg whites and oatmeal, and chicken and brown rice are all terrific options. Total calories should be about the same as in one of your "regular" meals. This will provide adequate fuel without bogging down your stomach.

Try to consume your pre-workout meal approximately two to three hours before training.[20] Allowing a couple of hours between the end of your meal and the onset of exercise will ensure that the majority of your meal is digested and will help to prevent gastric upset.

If you are attempting to gain mass, consider eating a large piece of fruit within a half hour of your workout. Due to a high concentration of fructose, fruits are low on the glycemic index.[21] This is significant because it keeps insulin levels stable, thereby preventing the potential for rebound hypoglycemia—a condition that can result in lightheadedness and fatigue.[22] At the same time, fruits provide a valuable source of fuel during exercise, improving your capacity to train.[23] Apples, pears, strawberries, and other low-glycemic fruits make excellent choices here.

Ideally, the piece of fruit should be combined with a whey-protein drink. Whey is a "fast-acting" protein, meaning it's rapidly absorbed into circulation.[24] This expedites the flow of amino acids to your muscles without having an appreciable impact on digestion. Aim for about one-tenth of a gram of whey per pound of body weight (e.g., a person weighing 150 pounds would need about 15 grams of whey) mixed in a water-based solution.

This is also a great time to have a cup of java (tea is great, too!). If you remember, caffeine acts on the sympathetic nervous system to increase catecholamine (epinephrine and norepinephrine) production.[25] Among their diverse functions, catecholamines mobilize fatty acids from adipocytes, allowing them to be utilized for energy. And since exercise increases caloric expenditure, the body can make immediate use of these fatty acids to fuel your muscles.

Caffeine also has a positive effect on exercise performance. With an abundance of fat in the blood, your body is less reliant on glycogen, glucose, and amino acids for energy, thereby delaying muscular fatigue. And by sparing glucose, your brain functions better (glucose is the primary fuel for your brain), allowing you to train with a greater degree of intensity. These benefits are present in activities lasting as little as sixty seconds or as long as two hours.[26]

WHAT TO EAT
DURING A WORKOUT

The most important nutrient to consume during training is water. As you work out, a large amount of water is lost through your sweat, breath, and perhaps urine. If these fluids aren't replenished, your exercise performance is bound to suffer. In fact, decrements in endurance and muscular strength can manifest after only a 2 percent reduction in hydration status.[27] When taken to the extreme, heat stroke or even circulatory collapse can occur. Clearly, exercise-induced dehydration must be avoided at all costs (see "Signs of Dehydration" below).

It is a mistake, however, to rely on thirst as an indicator for when to drink. Intense exercise inhibits the thirst sensors in your throat and gut; by the time you become thirsty, your body already is dehydrated.[28] This is compounded by the fact that, as you age, your thirst sensors become less and less sensitive.[29]

Signs of Dehydration

Dehydration can have detrimental effects on both your performance and health. Below are some of its more common symptoms. If you experience two or more of these symptoms while training, you might be dehydrated. If so, make sure to drink fluids immediately and take a little break from training until symptoms subside.

- Excessive thirst
- Dry mouth
- Chapped lips
- Dizziness
- Fatigue
- Headaches
- Irritability
- Lack of appetite

> ## Important Note
>
> Make sure to adjust the amount of calories you consume on training days so that it reflects your target daily intake. The foods consumed before, during, and after exercise aren't freebies! If you don't account for these additional calories, you'll end up gaining unwanted body fat. Remember, calories do count!

Therefore, during exercise, drink early and drink often. Consume 8 ounces of fluid immediately before your workout and then take small sips of water every fifteen or twenty minutes or so while training, varying the volume based on sweating rate.[30] This will ensure a continued state of hydration, keeping fluid balance intact.

As a rule, you don't need to consume any nutrients for workouts that last less than an hour.[31] Assuming you eat properly in the pre-workout period, your body has enough energy to last about sixty minutes without a decrease in performance. This should prevail regardless of how intensely you train.

For workouts exceeding an hour, it is beneficial to take in some additional nutrients. Liquids are preferable, here. A drink containing 30 to 60 grams of simple carbohydrate per hour helps to stimulate glycogen resynthesis, prevent muscle tissue breakdown, and sustain exercise performance.[32] Many of the commercial drinks are good choices and, as a bonus, often contain helpful electrolytes. For a cheaper alternative, an all-natural fruit juice (no sugar added) will do just fine.

If weight loss is your goal, be judicious with the amount of calories you consume at this time. Consider taking a few sips of your carb drink every ten minutes or so and only consume more if you really feel you need it. And remember that marathon workouts aren't necessary for achieving a terrific physique. It's the quality, not the quantity, of training that breeds results. Rarely should your sessions need to last more than sixty minutes unless you are training for a specific event.

WHAT TO EAT AFTER A WORKOUT

The postexercise meal is perhaps the most important meal of all. After an intense workout, your body is in a catabolic state. It has spent a good deal of its stored fuels (including glycogen and amino acids) and sustained damage to its muscle fibers. The good news is that this presents a window of opportunity for anabolism. By consuming the proper ratio of nutrients during this time, not only do you initiate the rebuilding of damaged tissue and energy reserves, but you do so in a supercompensated fashion that fosters improvements in both body composition and exercise performance.

One of the primary goals postexercise is to replenish glycogen stores. Because glucose is depleted during training, your muscles and liver are literally starved for carbohydrate. In response, several adaptations take place. For one, the GLUT4 transporters responsible for bringing glucose into muscle cells become much more active (see page 136 for a refresher on GLUT4). For another, your body stimulates the activity of glycogen synthase—the principal enzyme involved in promoting glycogen storage.[33] The combination of these factors facilitates the rapid uptake of glucose, allowing glycogen to be replenished at an accelerated rate.

Carbohydrates are best taken in liquid form and should come from simple, high-glycemic sources. This is one instance where it is beneficial to spike insulin levels. You see, insulin has both anabolic and anticatabolic functions, helping to increase protein synthesis, decrease protein breakdown, and shuttle glycogen into cells.[34] And this is one instance where elevated insulin won't promote increases in body fat. Because your muscles are in a depleted state, nutrients will tend to be used for lean tissue purposes rather than for fat storage.

In this case, a combination of glucose and fructose is ideal. In addition to promoting an insulin response, glucose is the primary source of muscle glycogen. Fructose, on the other hand, preferentially replenishes liver glycogen (glucose is of limited utility to the liver, a phenomenon called the "glucose paradox").[35] Thus, the two types of sugar work synergistically to restock the body's glycogen stores.

Grape and cranberry juices are generally good choices since they have a high ratio of glucose to fructose. A good starting point is to consume ½ gram of carbs per pound of ideal body weight.[36] Thus, if your goal weight is 150 pounds, then you'd consume 75 grams of carbs. If weight loss is your goal, cut this amount back to ¼ gram of carbs per pound of ideal body weight. Over time, assess how your body responds and modify the amount based on individual response.

The other main nutritional objective post-workout is to supply sufficient protein for tissue repair. If protein intake is inadequate following training, recuperation is shortchanged and results are compromised.

Protein should preferably be in the form of a high-quality protein powder. The idea is to bathe your muscles in amino acids, providing them with the raw materials to facilitate recovery. The upshot is significant: When amino acids are consumed following training, protein synthesis is increased more than threefold over fasting conditions.[37] In this way, muscle fibers are built back up so they're stronger than before.

A fast-acting protein such as whey works best. Because it is rapidly assimilated, whey reaches your muscles quickly, thereby expediting repair. And since your muscles are primed for anabolism, virtually all of the protein will be utilized for rebuilding with little wastage. Aim for ¼ gram of protein per pound of ideal body weight, mixing the powder directly into your post-workout drink.

As in the pre-workout meal, it is best to refrain from consuming fats following your workout. Since fat slows gastric emptying, it delays the time that glucose and amino acids can enter the bloodstream and be used by the body. And if nutrients don't reach your muscles in a timely fashion, results will suffer.

Caffeinated beverages should also be avoided during this period. Caffeine interferes with postexercise insulin action, thereby impairing your body's ability to replenish glycogen stores and utilize protein for muscular repair.[38] Hence, wait at least a couple of hours after your workout before indulging in that cup of coffee or tea.

Ideally, you should consume your post-workout meal as soon as possible after training. The quicker you feed your body, the more it sops up nutrients and utilizes

Summary of the Look Great Naked Diet Protocol for Exercise

1. Consume a meal containing a low-glycemic carbohydrate and lean protein source about two to three hours before training. Keep fat consumption to a minimum.
2. If weight gain is desired, have a large piece of fruit and some whey protein (amounting to one-tenth of a gram per pound of body weight) within a half hour of training.
3. To maximize fat loss, consume a cup of coffee or tea before training.
4. Consume 8 ounces of fluid immediately prior to your workout and then take small sips of water every fifteen or twenty minutes or so while training.
5. For workouts lasting more than an hour, consume a drink containing 30 to 60 grams of simple carbohydrates (such as a fruit juice or sports drink).
6. Following training, consume a drink containing high-glycemic carbohydrate (such as grape juice or cranberry juice) and a high-quality protein powder. Generally, carbohydrate should amount to about ½ gram per pound of body weight (¼ gram per pound of body weight for those seeking to maximize fat loss) and protein should amount to about ¼ gram per pound of body weight.

them for repair. Since blood flow is increased from the exercise bout, the delivery of protein and carbs is enhanced, resulting in greater muscle protein synthesis.[39]

But even if you are unable to consume your post-workout meal immediately upon cessation of training, all is not lost. The window of opportunity lasts for at least a couple of hours following exercise (albeit in somewhat of a diminished state) so just make sure you take in the specified nutrients as soon as you can. Don't allow this opportunity to slip away.

NUTRITIONAL KNOW-HOW

PART FOUR

CHAPTER 11

Eating Healthy When Eating Out

Nothing can derail your diet more than dining out. After all, it's fairly easy to eat properly when you're in the comfort of your own home. You can simply discard all the "bad" foods from your pantry or refrigerator, removing any temptation to binge on fattening foods. But go out to a restaurant or a party and all bets are off. Studies show a high correlation between restaurant frequency and increased body fatness.[1]

Clearly, the best way to stay lean is to prepare all your food yourself. But in the real world, this isn't always possible. The average American eats away from home four days a week, accounting for 32 percent of daily energy intake[2]. Breakfast meetings, business lunches, dinner parties—in today's society, dining out is an unavoidable fact of life.

Fortunately, with the proper approach, it's possible to maintain a healthy nutritional regimen, even when you're away from home. By adhering to the following protocol, you can stay the course and maintain a terrific physique—regardless of where you may be dining.

PASS ON THE BREAD

At the beginning of a meal, it is customary in most restaurants to put a basket full of bread on your table. Unfortunately, this practice starts things off on the wrong foot. Each slice of bread can contain upward of a couple of hundred calories. Put on a slab of butter and you'll double this amount. Worse, restaurant breads are usually made from finely ground white flour—a glycemic nightmare that spikes insulin levels. Your best bet is to ask to have the bread basket taken away so it won't be a temptation. At most, limit your consumption to a slice or two, dipping in extra virgin olive oil rather than smearing with butter.

HOLD THE SOUP

As an appetizer, soup is king. Virtually every restaurant has a "soup du jour." Soups are so popular that they're often included as a part of lunch and dinner specials. However, unknown to many, soups are loaded with sodium. Not only does sodium elevate blood pressure levels, but it also causes your body to retain water (see Chapter 7 for details). When too much sodium is ingested, fluid is drawn out of the cells and into the body's free spaces, resulting in a bloated appearance. Your feet and hands swell, your face becomes puffy, and water accumulates beneath your skin—not a desirable condition for someone trying to stay lean.

To avoid this fate, it's best to refrain from soups, choosing an alternate appetizer instead. In most cases, there are plenty of sodium-free options available. If not, pass on the appetizer altogether; there's no rule that says you must have a multi-course meal.

SKIP THE DRINKS

By now, the detriments of alcohol consumption should be readily apparent (they were discussed at length in Chapter 9). But just to recap in case you missed it: Alcohol promotes body-fat storage. It is calorically dense, containing more than seven calories per gram (as opposed to carbs and protein, which have four). Worse, many drinks are mixed with high-calorie items such as whole milk, soda, and juice. For the most part, alcoholic beverages provide little or no nutritional value. They are "empty calories" that serve only to pack on unwanted pounds. Consequently, try to avoid alcohol when you are out socially. To quench your thirst, stick with water or club soda. If you must indulge, a wine spritzer or lite beer is your best bet.

HAVE IT DRY

Greasy, fried meals are the rule rather than the exception at most restaurants. They often baste meats, veggies, and other foods with butter. Or they'll cook with an unsaturated vegetable oil that, under high heat, becomes a rancid, toxic trans fat. Don't blame the chef, though. Butter and oil make foods taste better and, since taste is a restaurant's primary concern, they are used in abundance during cooking. However, this can add an enormous amount of calories to a meal and clog your arteries with a profusion of unhealthy saturated and trans fats.

Realize that foods don't have to be greasy in order to be palatable. By using the right combination of spices, caloric balance can be maintained without sacrificing flavor. Hence, rather than opting for something fried, order your foods broiled, steamed, or baked. To ensure that no additional fat is added, ask to have everything prepared "dry." And if the waiter gives you a hard time about this, just tell him that you're allergic to butter and oil. I guarantee he'll acquiesce and honor your request.

GET IT ON THE SIDE

The secret of many recipes is in the sauce. Vodka, Alfredo, and other cream-based mixtures help to give foods their distinct flavor. However, these sauces can turn an otherwise healthy meal into an all-out fat-fest (think fillet of sole soaked in tartar sauce or salad greens smothered with bleu cheese dressing!). To keep calories in line, ask that any sauce or dressing be served on the side. Then, if you wish, lightly dip your food in the sauce—just enough to add some flavor. Remember: when it comes to sauce, less is more!

EAT YOUR VEGGIES

Your mother was right: vegetables really are a nutritional panacea. Green vegetables, in particular, are an ideal food. They are replete in vitamins and minerals, devoid of saturated fat, and extremely low in calories (a pound of broccoli, for example, contains only 120 calories!). But there's an even more important reason why vegetables should be consumed: they suppress hunger. Because of their bulk, they take up a large amount of space in the stomach, helping to fill you up without filling you out. In effect, they are like green water—you can eat as much as you want without the fear of gaining weight. This is especially important in a restaurant setting, where a multitude of menu choices tend to encourage binge eating. So make sure you have a big salad as an appetizer and some greens as part of dinner. Better yet, get a double serving of veggies with your entrée instead of a starch; this in itself will lop several hundred calories from your meal.

OPT FOR FRUIT

Chocolate cheesecake, crème brûlée, tiramisù . . . there's no doubt that desserts tend to be the most fattening of all foods. While they may taste great, the great majority are chock-full of sugar and saturated fat—a lethal combination in terms of promoting weight gain. Here is where you must exert a great deal of willpower. Passing up on sumptuous sweets requires the ability to forgo instant gratification for long-term benefit—not an easy task. Fruits are the perfect alternative. They are rich in fiber, plentiful in vitamins and minerals, and low on the glycemic scale (they don't cause a spike in insulin levels). And, best of all, they taste great! Even if it's not on the dessert menu, a fruit plate can almost always be made to order; all you have to do is ask.

BANISH THE BUFFET

The concept of an all-you-can-eat buffet sounds great, right? Wrong—at least not if you're trying to keep your body fit! A buffet puts you in a position where you're bound to overindulge. This has been demonstrated time and again in research studies. When allowed to eat at will (called an *ad libitum diet*), people consistently eat more than when food is doled out in measured portions. Hence, try to steer clear of all-you-can-eat restaurants whenever possible. If you simply can't avoid it, try to fill up on salads at the beginning of your meal and load up on veggies for your entrée. And once you've eaten your main course, don't go back for seconds!

CHAPTER 12

Preparing for the Big Event

Okay, you've got it all together—you're training hard, eating right, and living a fitness lifestyle. And your body is beginning to respond. You've lost inches off your waist and have started to see definition in places where you didn't even think you had muscles. All is going great, but you want more. You've got a big-time event coming up shortly and you really want to look your absolute best.

Every so often, a specific occasion arises that drives a person to pull out all the stops. It might be a wedding, a pool party, a high school reunion, or even a fitness or physique competition. You'll be in some sort of revealing outfit in front of a group of people, probably having to pose for an endless stream of photographs. Perhaps you'll even be captured on video or, gasp, appear on TV!

If you are faced with such a situation, a specific nutritional regimen called carb depletion/carb loading is in order. The theory behind the strategy is simple. When carbs are drastically depleted, your body is forced to utilize all of its stored glycogen for energy. Glycogen, if you remember, is the stored form of carbohydrate. It is abundant in the liver and muscles, providing a source of short-term energy. Why is this important? Well, glycogen is hydrophilic (it attracts water). For each gram of glycogen, the body stores approximately 3 grams of water.[1]

Now here's where nutritional science comes in. By depleting glycogen, water is simultaneously excreted from your muscles and liver; the more glycogen you deplete, the more your body "dries out." Then, as soon as carbs are reintroduced, your muscles and liver rapidly take up glucose in order to replenish glycogen stores. More important, any water held subcutaneously (beneath the skin) is drawn into the cells along with the glycogen. If you do it right, your physique appears lean and hard, with full, shapely muscles that really stand out.

Realize, though, that a carb depletion/carb loading scheme is most effective when you are at or near your ideal body composition. It is not intended to be a quick-fix weight-loss program. Rather, it is a means to optimize your physique for a specific event (and shouldn't be used as a long-term strategy). If you are carrying a lot of body fat, the visible effects of the program will be seriously compromised.

Ideally, the diet should commence one week prior to the affair. For best results, adhere to the following protocols.

THE CARB DEPLETION PHASE

Carb depletion should begin seven days before the event and last for a total of three days. Hence, assuming the event is on a Saturday, carb depletion should begin on Sunday and last through Tuesday. The goal here is to dissipate all glycogen from the muscles and liver by the end of this phase.

Nutrition

The first step in the process is to drastically cut carbohydrate intake. A good rule of thumb is to limit carbs to no more than about 10 percent of total calories. The carbs that you do consume should be nutrient dense and preferably contain some fiber to maintain regularity. It is advisable to ingest these carbs early in the day. Since glucose is the primary source of fuel for the brain and central nervous system, this will help to keep energy levels up. Oatmeal and bran cereals make excellent choices, as do other unrefined grains. Green vegetables also are an important part of the mix and, since they are extremely low in caloric composition, can be consumed in abundance.

To make up for the reduction in carbs, approximately 50 percent of your calories should come from dietary fat. If desired, it's okay to eat foods high in saturated fat (such as bacon, hamburger, and hard cheeses). Don't worry about any health consequences: the time frame is too short for intake of these products to have any negative effects on your well-being. Of course, mono- and polyunsaturated sources (such as seeds, oils, and nuts) are even better options and, if possible, should make up the majority of fat consumption.

An excellent fat-based alternative is medium-chain triglycerides (MCTs). MCTs are a special type of fat. They have a unique molecular structure that allows them to bypass the body's usual fat-storage mechanisms. Rather than breaking down into fatty acids, MCTs are transported directly into the liver where they are rapidly converted into an instant energy source. Due to this occurrence, the body prefers to utilize them for short-term fuel.[2] So by including MCTs during carb depletion, you can help to maintain elevated energy levels without risking unwanted fat deposition. MCTs come in liquid form and can be added directly to foods and beverages. They can be purchased in most health food stores. Just make sure you don't consume them directly before exercise as they can cause gastrointestinal discomfort, which can reduce performance.[3]

Protein should make up the balance of the diet, equating to roughly 40 percent of total calories. Although some people cut back on protein intake when carb depleting in order to minimize gluconeogenesis (the conversion of protein to glucose), this thinking is decidedly misguided. If protein intake is inadequate, the body is apt to cannibalize its muscle tissue for fuel—especially during times of caloric restriction. Only by keeping protein intake high will you attenuate any potential muscle loss. As far as gluconeogenesis, it's really a nonissue: the amount of protein conversion to glucose is relatively insignificant at this point and has little effect on glycogen resynthesis.

Exercise

During the carb depletion phase, you should work out every day, training all the major muscles of your body each time you exercise. Muscles lack an enzyme (called glucose-6-phosphatase) that allows glucose to be utilized in other bodily tissues. Since glucose is so important for muscular action, this is nature's way of preserving muscle glycogen for future use. Consequently, the only way to completely expend all of your muscle glycogen is by training the entire body.

As far as the mode of exercise, you can either choose to weight train or perform aerobics. If you decide to weight train, it's best to perform one exercise for each major muscle group. Very high reps (twenty-five or more per set) are advisable, execut-

Table 12.1

PROTOCOLS FOR THE CARB DEPLETION PHASE	
NUTRIENT	**PERCENTAGE OF TOTAL CALORIES**
Carbohydrate	10
Protein	40
Fat	50

ing the movements in a slow, controlled fashion. It isn't necessary, though, to train with a great deal of intensity during this period. The concept is to facilitate glycogen depletion, not to develop your muscles. Consequently, you should terminate each set just short of reaching muscular fatigue. One or two sets per muscle group will do the trick—any more and you risk overtraining.

If you prefer, light cardiovascular activity is an acceptable alternative to weight training. Again, make sure to utilize exercises that work the entire body to ensure glycogen is fully depleted. The treadmill or bike alone simply won't do. You also need to incorporate an upper-body aerobic movement such as rowing, elliptical training, or cross-country skiing. Keep intensity relatively low, staying in a range of about 60 to 70 percent of maximal heart rate.

It's important to realize that by the end of the three-day depletion phase, your body won't look like you want it to. Your muscles will be flat and your face will be drawn. What's more, you'll probably feel a little weak and lethargic. Don't worry! Once you carb load, all of these effects will be reversed. Provided you stick with the protocols, all will be well by that special day.

THE CARB LOADING PHASE

Carb loading should begin on the fourth day and last for two more days. So for the same Saturday event, carb loading will take place on Wednesday and Thursday. You now want to replenish all of your glycogen stores, achieving a phenomenon known as glycogen supercompensation.[4]

During this phase, jack up carbohydrate intake to around 60 percent of total calories. Consume mostly starchy brown carbs such as brown rice, yams, oatmeal, and other whole grains. Vegetables should be kept to a minimum, as they will fill you up without doing much to enhance glycogen uptake. To ensure maximal absorption, spread out carb intake throughout the day, eating small amounts with every meal.

Dietary fat–particularly of the saturated variety–must be avoided at all costs. Due to the high carbohydrate consumption, insulin levels will be consistently elevated during this phase. If you remember, insulin is a storage hormone and turns on various mechanisms that promote the deposition of body fat. Hence, when excess fats are consumed in conjunction with high levels of insulin, the potential for fat storage is significantly increased.[5] You should, therefore, consume only essential fatty acids (such as flaxseed or fish oil) and keep intake to about 10 percent of calories.

Protein will make up the balance of calories (approximately 30 percent of total caloric intake). As opposed to the depletion phase, you now must stay clear of bacon, cheeses, and creams since they are extremely high in fat. Stick with lean protein sources, such as white meat poultry, egg whites, and protein powders instead.

You should refrain from performing any type of exercise during this period. While you might be inclined to believe that training right up until the end is beneficial, it's not. In fact, it's actually counterproductive. Working out only serves to deplete the very glycogen stores that you're trying to replenish. You'll end up looking flat and stringy–not full and hard. Hence, resist any temptation to go to the gym, regardless of the psychological urge to train.

You can, however, "pose" your muscles (hold them in a contracted position for twenty to thirty seconds at a time) during carb loading. If you are preparing for a physique-oriented competition, this technique is especially beneficial. It will help to increase your muscular endurance and allow you to hold your poses for extended periods of time.

Table 12.2

PROTOCOLS FOR THE CARB LOADING PHASE	
NUTRIENT	**PERCENTAGE OF TOTAL CALORIES**
Carbohydrate	60
Protein	30
Fat	10

FINAL PREPARATION

Finally, on the last day before the event, carb intake should be adjusted according to your appearance—increased if you look flat or reduced if you look bloated. If you've nailed it on the head, you should be right on for your special occasion!

On the "big day," you should again assess your physique. While your ability to significantly change your appearance is limited at this point, minor adjustments can still be made. If all is well, stick with small portions of dried fruit right up until the time of the event.

A final note: People respond differently to a carb deplete/carb load scheme. It is therefore beneficial to experiment with this technique several months before your event. This is particularly important if you are entering a physique-oriented competition. If you're going to be judged on your appearance in comparison to others, you certainly don't want to tempt fate. Once you go through the regimen once or twice, you'll be comfortable with how your body reacts and be able to make adjustments based on your individual response.

CHAPTER 13

The Scoop on Supplements

With more than $16 billion a year spent on vitamins, herbs, and other compounds, supplements are big business. And it's no wonder. The allure of a magic pill—one that miraculously melts away fat, builds muscle, or restores vim and vigor—is hard to resist. And herein lies the problem: Consumers are so enamored with this premise that they're easy prey to fast-talking snake oil salesmen who promise an easy way to a great body.

For decades, the Food and Drug Administration (FDA) helped to keep things honest. They served as a watchdog over the supplement industry, certifying that products were safe and wholesome, and that their labeling was accurate and not misleading. In order for a supplement to pass FDA standards, it had to undergo stringent safety and efficacy testing. Supplements that weren't up to snuff never made it onto store shelves.

All of this changed in 1994 when, in an attempt to ensure that consumers had ready access to potentially healthful supplements, Congress passed the Dietary Supplements Health and Education Act (DSHEA). The gist of this legislation provides that as long as a substance found in nature doesn't claim to treat or cure a disease, it isn't subject to regulation by the FDA. In effect, it's now up to the government to prove that a particular supplement is unsafe[1]—a difficult proposition, to say the least.

Fast-forward to today: There are currently more than 30,000 dietary supplements available in the United States with more than 1,000 new ones being introduced each year. You can find them everywhere, from health food stores to pharmacies to super-markets to gas stations. Whether you're a preadolescent or an octogenarian, man or woman, Caucasian or African-American, the consumption of supplements crosses all demographic bounds. Clearly, from the standpoint of facilitating consumer access, DSHEA has accomplished its mission.

But with the good also comes the bad: Without the benefit of FDA supervision, the supplement industry is now rife with deceit and fraud. Seizing on an opportunity to make a quick buck, legions of unscrupulous hucksters have entered the market, peddling quick-fix solutions with little or no physiologic basis. It's almost impossible to turn on the TV or flip through a magazine without seeing glitzy advertisements and infomercials for bogus products such as "Exercise in a Bottle" or "Ultimate Fat Trapper." The onus is now on consumers to make educated choices and separate supplementation fact from fiction—something that most are not informed enough to do.

WHAT WORKS, WHAT DOESN'T

Let me say this up front: You don't need supplements to achieve a terrific body—anyone that tells you otherwise undoubtedly has a hidden agenda. Upward of 95 percent of your results are a function of proper diet, exercise, and rest. Provided you eat right, train hard, and allow for adequate recuperation, you'll look great naked—guaranteed.

That said, if you want to take your body from the 95 percent threshold up to its maximum, supplements can be beneficial. When properly utilized, they provide an extra boost that helps you attain your personal best.

At elite levels of sport, supplementation is highly advantageous, perhaps even crucial. Here, small differences in performance and/or body composition can mean the difference between winning and losing a competition. By giving you that slight edge, the right supplement regimen can very well push you over the top.

Unfortunately, the vast majority of supplements have little, if any, efficacy (at least in otherwise healthy individuals). For example, consider the popular supplement L-carnitine, a compound abundant in meats, poultry, and dairy products. Although not an essential nutrient, a deficiency of L-carnitine can diminish your ability to burn fat. This is because its primary function is to transport fatty acids across the mitochondrial membrane so they can be used for fuel. Without an adequate supply of L-carnitine, fatty acids cannot be properly oxidized and fat burning comes to a halt.

Here's where clever marketing practices come into play. Claiming that increased amounts of dietary L-carnitine allow more fat to be delivered to the mitochondria for oxidation, supplement companies promote L-carnitine as an aid to fat burning and include it as an ingredient in many fat-burning supplements and performance enhancers. Sounds like a reasonable theory, right? Well, as is often the case, theory doesn't always translate into practice. In healthy individuals, L-carnitine can be readily synthesized in the body from the amino acids lysine and methionine. Provided you take in adequate protein, the risk of deficiency is virtually nonexistent. And in the absence of a deficiency, L-carnitine supplementation has no effect on fat loss or athletic performance.[2,3] The evidence is clear: While it's true that L-carnitine is integral to cellular metabolism, taking supraphysiological doses beyond what your body requires is of no additional benefit.

My intent here isn't to single out L-carnitine. Numerous other supplements are similarly marketed under false pretenses. Chromium and vanadyl sulfate come to mind immediately but there are many, many more. The bottom line is that, when it comes to supplementation, you need to heed the old Latin saying: *caveat emptor*—let the buyer beware.

So how do you determine which supplements to take and which to avoid? The decision comes down to cost/benefit; namely, do the benefits outweigh the costs? And cost is not just a function of money; the potential adverse effects on health must also be considered. There is a common misperception among consumers that natural compounds are harmless. Supplement companies play on this perceived notion, marketing products with the words "herbal" and/or "all natural" emblazoned on the label. But just because a supplement is natural doesn't necessarily mean it's safe for human consumption. Cyanide, arsenic, and hemlock are natural substances that can be lethal, even in small doses. Opium, hashish, and cocaine are also natural compounds . . . get the point?

Realize, too, that herbs can have undesirable interactions with certain drugs. For example, ginkgo biloba extract, used for improving cognitive function, can increase the risk of bleeding when used with blood thinners and antiplatelet agents; St.-John's-wort, promoted as a treatment for depression, may interfere with the actions of monoamine oxidase (MAO) inhibitors; and ginseng, widely used as an energy booster, has been implicated as a cause of decreased response to warfarin.[4]

When buying supplements, make sure they are from a reputable manufacturer.

Since the industry is all but unregulated, quality can vary significantly between brands. Laboratory analysis has found a wide variation in what is on the label and what is in the bottle. For example, some products contain less than 10 percent of the claimed amount of the active ingredient. Others contain banned pesticides, undeclared heavy metals, prescription drugs, and other potentially dangerous substances[5] (one brand of chromium picolinate was found to be contaminated with hexavalent chromium, the toxic form of the mineral most notably popularized in the movie *Erin Brockovich*!). Check out the Resources section for a list of Web sites that provide independent testing of many of the most popular supplements.

Now that we've covered the basics, it's time to get down to specifics. From a body-composition perspective, supplements can be broken down into two separate groups: vitamins and minerals, and muscle builders. Let's discuss each of these groups in detail. (I will cover only those supplements that have proven to be efficacious.)

VITAMINS AND MINERALS

For generations, vitamins and minerals were touted as wonder supplements, heralded for curing everything from hair loss to night blindness. While we now know these claims to be greatly exaggerated, it doesn't diminish the fact that adequate intake of vitamins and minerals is imperative for maintaining a fit, healthy body. They facilitate energy transfer, prevent disease, and act as coenzymes to assist in many chemical reactions. A deficiency in any of these micronutrients can lead to severe illness. For instance, a lack of vitamin B_6 results in pellagra; too little vitamin D leads to rickets; and a thiamine deficiency causes beriberi.

Take Your Multivitamin

In order to address vitamin and mineral needs, the United States government developed a Recommended Dietary Allowance (RDA) for each micronutrient. These guidelines set a minimum nutrient intake, below which you can expect to contract disease. The RDAs have been considered the "gold standard" for micronutrient intake ever since.

To ensure that you meet the RDAs for all vitamins and minerals, I highly recommend that you take a supplemental multivitamin/mineral complex. Depending on your choice of foods and total caloric intake, there is always the possibility that you might not get enough of a specific micronutrient (calcium and folate can be especially difficult to acquire through normal dietary means). Taking a multi serves as an "insurance policy," helping to prevent against any deficiencies. And there's really no downside: The cost is minimal and any micronutrients not utilized by your body are simply excreted in your urine without ill effect.

Antioxidants

A special class of micronutrients called antioxidants should be supplemented on an individual basis. There is a large body of scientific evidence showing that antioxidants are required in much larger amounts than other vitamins and minerals—far in excess of what is prescribed in the RDA guidelines. It's important to realize that the RDAs were established to prevent deficiencies, not to improve overall health and wellness, and antioxidants have additional health-related benefits above and beyond their basic functions.

So what's so special about these compounds? Well, antioxidants are the body's scavengers. They help to defend against damage caused by free radicals—unstable molecules that can injure healthy cells and tissues. Millions of these gremlins are produced each day during the normal course of respiration. The main culprit: oxygen. Every time you breathe, oxygen uptake causes free-radical production. Environmental factors such as pollutants, smoke, and certain chemicals also contribute to their formation. If left unchecked, they can wreak havoc on your physique and cause a multitude of ailments including arthritis, cardiovascular disease, dementia, and cancer.[6]

Here's a short course in how the process works: Your body is made up of billions of cells held together by a series of electronic bonds. These bonds are arranged in pairs so that one electron balances the other. However, in response to various occurrences (such as oxygen consumption), a molecule can lose one of its electron pairs, making it an unstable free radical. The free radical then tries to replace its lost electron by stealing one from another molecule. This sets up a chain reaction where the second molecule becomes a free radical and attacks a third molecule, which becomes a free radical and then attacks a fourth molecule and so on.

To prevent rampant free-radical production, your body has a sophisticated internal antioxidant system. Various antioxidant enzymes combine with antioxidants from the foods you eat to help keep free radicals at bay. But when free-radical activity reaches a critical level, the system can become overwhelmed, causing extensive damage to cellular tissues.

Compounding matters, your antioxidant system tends to degenerate with age.

Antioxidant enzymes such as superoxide dismutase and glutathione reductase become less responsive over time.[7] These age-related changes make cells even more susceptible to free-radical-induced damage.

Although antioxidants can be obtained through dietary means, it's virtually impossible to consume adequate quantities from food sources alone. For example, you'd have to drink eleven glasses of orange juice in order to get the needed amount of vitamin C or 8 pounds of spinach to get the needed amount of vitamin E! And since it has been shown that, at low doses (even above RDA guidelines), antioxidants don't provide adequate protection against infirmity, supplementation isn't an option—it's a necessity.[8] Given that side effects are virtually nonexistent at prescribed levels, there is very little risk and great potential reward.

For the active person, antioxidant supplementation is of particular importance.[9] Due to increased oxygen consumption, free-radical production skyrockets during exercise (by as much as twentyfold over resting levels) and the body's internal defense system is unable to cope.[10] If left unchecked, this results in an inflammation of muscle tissue, impairing muscular function and slowing recovery.[11]

While there are dozens of known antioxidants, two are absolutely indispensable: vitamins E and C. These vitamins are partners in defense; they have a synergistic relationship, working together so that their combined effect is greater than the sum of their individual actions.[12]

Vitamin E (alpha-tocopherol) is perhaps the most heralded of all antioxidants. Because of its fat-soluble nature, vitamin E exerts its influence on the outer part of the cell (i.e., the cell membrane). A large body of evidence shows that it is cardioprotective, helping to reduce arteriosclerotic plaques that are implicated in heart disease and stroke. The now-famous Cambridge study showed that, in sufficient doses, vitamin E supplementation dramatically reduces the rate of mortality and morbidity in cardiac patients, with beneficial effects apparent even after a year of treatment.[13] There also is some evidence that vitamin E helps to prevent various forms of cancer, especially in the prostate.[14] Between 400 and 800 IU is recommended for optimal health.[15] It is best to consume a natural derivative of alpha-tocopherol; the synthetic form is not as well absorbed into tissues.[16]

Vitamin C (ascorbic acid), on the other hand, is water soluble and therefore scavenges the plasma. Like vitamin E, it helps to reduce cardiovascular risk by preventing lipid peroxidation.[17] In addition, there is mounting evidence that it acts as an anticarcinogen, protecting against cancers of the bladder, breast, cervix, colon, esophagus, lungs, pancreas, prostate, salivary gland, stomach, and lymphatic system.[18] Less clear is its ability to enhance immune function. Although some swear by the fact that megadoses can cure various ailments (such as the common cold), supporting evidence is still equivocal in this regard. Daily doses of 600 to 1,000 mg are recommended to achieve a therapeutic effect.[19]

Two other compounds, coenzyme Q_{10} and alpha-lipoic acid, should also be considered important supplements. Not only are they powerful antioxidants in their own right, but they also help to regenerate vitamins E and C[20,21] (antioxidants become inactive after they quench a free radical). In this way, they bolster your body's defense system, providing the ultimate in free-radical prevention.

Numerous other antioxidants including selenium, polyphenols, and carotenoids also are involved in quenching free radicals. Research on the efficacy of supplementing these "ancillary" compounds is less impressive, though. The decision to take them in supplemental form is a judgment call.

As a rule, it is best to consume supplemental vitamins and minerals in conjunction with a meal. The absorption of micronutrients is improved when they are taken with food. This also improves gastrointestinal tolerance of the supplement.

Table 13.1 lists some of the most important antioxidants and their prescribed dosages. I highly recommend supplementing with vitamin C, vitamin E, coenzyme Q_{10}, and alpha-lipoic acid. The other antioxidants can be taken if desired but should not be considered essential.

Table 13.1

ANTIOXIDANTS AND RECOMMENDED DOSAGES	
NUTRIENT	**SUGGESTED DOSAGE**
Vitamin C	800 mg
Vitamin E	600 IU
Coenzyme Q_{10}	50 mg
Alpha-lipoic acid	100 mg
Polyphenols	50 mg
Lycopene	10 mg
Selenium	200 mcg

MUSCLE BUILDERS

Of all the muscle-building supplements, none has received more attention than creatine. From bodybuilders to professional athletes to Olympic competitors, creatine is used at every level of sport. And with good reason: It's the only compound that actually works in practice.

Before getting into the nitty-gritty, a little background info is in order. Creatine is a nutrient synthesized from three amino acids: arginine, glycine, and methionine. Approximately 95 percent of your creatine supply is stored in muscle tissue, with the balance located primarily in your heart, brain, and, in men, the testes. Its primary function is to power your muscles, particularly during movements that are quick and explosive in nature. This is accomplished largely through its interaction with the high-energy compound adenosine triphosphate (ATP). During intense exercise, ATP serves as the initial fuel for muscular contractions. But there is only enough ATP available to fuel about ten seconds worth of activity. Here's where creatine comes into play. It helps to regenerate ATP, thereby allowing you to continue training in an intense fashion for another twenty seconds or so.

Given its importance in muscular function, the benefits of maintaining ample amounts of bodily creatine should be obvious. Supplementation has proven to be effective in this regard. By allowing larger stores of creatine to build up in muscle tissue, you are able to exercise longer and harder. This is especially beneficial during weight training. With more creatine available, you can squeeze out a few extra reps per set.[22] And this increased training capacity translates into an ability to build more muscle.

Creatine also increases muscular growth by promoting cellular hydration.[23] You see, when creatine is stored in muscles, it pulls in water along with it. This causes the muscles to swell, which stimulates protein synthesis and inhibits protein breakdown—the basis for muscular development.[24] Better yet, since creatine is primarily stored in fast-twitch fibers—the ones with the greatest potential for growth—its muscle-building effects are heightened.[25]

Realize, though, creatine is no wonder supplement. Despite the lofty claims made by some individuals, it won't give you "steroidlike" results. Muscular gains are less than exceptional, with most users adding no more than a few of pounds of lean body weight.[26] From a performance perspective, average improvements are relatively modest—you're not going to double the amount of weight you squat or curl. If you're expecting it to miraculously transform your body, you'll end up being very disappointed.

Furthermore, creatine doesn't work for everybody. About 30 percent of the population are considered "nonresponders" who achieve little or no benefit from supplementation. This seems to be dependent on the body's internal creatine stores.[27] You see, only a limited amount of creatine can be stored in the muscles (approximately 120 grams for an average-sized male). Once these stores are full, any excess is of no utility and is excreted from the body through the urine. Thus, if you're one of those people who have naturally high amounts of muscle creatine, supplementation will be fruitless.

Still and all, there isn't much of a downside to taking creatine. It does promote some muscle growth in the majority of people and is virtually free from side effects.[28,29] (Other than some isolated reports of muscle cramping, no other symptoms have been associated with its use.) So assuming money is not an issue, creatine is definitely worth a try if you want to maximize muscle mass.

Creatine is traditionally taken in two phases: A loading phase (to thoroughly saturate the muscles with creatine) followed by a maintenance phase (to keep creatine stores full). Standard advice is to take 20 to 30 grams for the first week (spread out over four or five servings) and then 2 grams thereafter for maintenance.[30] I've found that taking a daily dose of five days over the course of one month serves the same purpose as loading without the hassle of frequent consumption. And don't think that increasing intake above recommended levels will be of any additional benefit. Remember, there is a definable upper limit to the body's capacity to store creatine in muscle; above this limit, further supplementation simply results in its excretion.[31]

Ideally, creatine should be consumed with a high-glycemic carbohydrate drink such as grape juice or cranberry juice.[32] The associated insulin response helps to drive creatine into your muscles, maximizing its storage. And stick with pure creatine monohydrate. There is no evidence that gimmicky variants such as effervescent or liquid creatine have any additional benefits, and they are much more expensive.

CHAPTER 14

The Biggest Myths in Nutrition and Fat Loss

MYTH: Women shouldn't lift weights because they'll bulk up.

In the not-so-distant past, it was considered taboo for women to lift weights. Gyms were basically dark, dingy, basement-oriented clubs dominated by men. The vast majority of women perceived them as seedy, sweat-ridden dungeons that were primarily inhabited by brainless "muscleheads." What's more, there was insufficient information and knowledge about the potential benefits of exercise for women; essentially, strength training was thought of only as a means to grow big and bulky, with little other utility. The prevailing belief was that it decreased femininity—that it in effect "masculinized" the female physique.

Fortunately, times have changed. The majority of women now understand that strength training is the key to a firm, shapely body. Women now make up more than half of all gym memberships, and recent statistics show that almost a quarter of the female population lifts weights on a regular basis.

However, to a great extent, women's training remains an enigma. While realizing that lifting weights is beneficial, women still tend to have an innate fear that it will bulk them up. Consequently, they often train halfheartedly, using extremely "light" weights that don't sufficiently tax the neuromuscular system. It's no wonder, then, that most fail to achieve adequate results.

In truth, it's extremely difficult for a woman to develop large muscles. The main reason: a lack of testosterone. Testosterone is a hormone that's secreted by the testes (in males) and, to a lesser extent, by the ovaries (in females). It has two main functions: First, testosterone is *androgenic* (i.e., masculinizing); it promotes male-oriented characteristics such as the growth of facial and body hair, male-pattern baldness, and deepening of the voice.[1] Second, testosterone is *anabolic* (building); through a complex process, it interacts at the cellular level with muscle tissue to increase protein synthesis[2]–the primary stimulus for initiating muscular growth. Hence, there is a direct relationship between testosterone and muscle mass: the more testosterone you secrete, the greater your propensity to pack on muscle.

On average, women produce only about one-tenth the amount of testosterone as their male counterparts[3]; this is nature's way of preserving "femininity." As a result, it's virtually impossible for women to add a significant amount of muscular bulk to their frame. Without an anabolic stimulus, muscle tissue simply has no impetus to hypertrophy and muscular growth remains modest, even at advanced levels of training.

Given the upside, strength training should be an essential component in any nutritional program, whether you're a man or a woman. By helping to maintain, or even increase, resting metabolic rate, it allows you to slim down in a safe, effective manner. And it even helps to lower your set point so that you stay lean over the long haul!

MYTH: You should eat according to your blood type.

The theory that your blood type should dictate eating patterns, popularized by Dr. Peter D'Adamo in his book *Eat Right 4 Your Type,* is one of today's biggest nutritional crazes. Dr. D'Adamo puts forth the hypothesis that your blood type is a product of evolution and, because of the evolutionary process, impacts the way in which your body responds to various foods. Here is a brief synopsis: Type O's are the "original" blood type and consequently thrive on the high-protein/low-carbohydrate diets of cavemen; type A's descended from farmers (around 25,000 B.C.), so they respond best to high-carb/low-protein vegetarian diets; type B's trace their ancestry to nomads (emerging about 15,000 years ago) and should therefore eat a mixed diet; and type AB's (evolving within the past 1,000 years) are an amalgam of types A and B, allowing them the leeway to consume a combination of the two diets.

The basic premise of the diet revolves around food-based proteins called lectins and their ability to cause agglutination (a reaction in which particles suspended in a liquid collect into clumps). According to proponents of the blood type diet, the lectins contained in certain foods cause a host of unwanted reactions in people who are not genetically suited to consume these foods; if you don't eat right for your type, bad things are bound to happen.

Alternatively, by eating in a manner that does coincide with your blood type, proponents of this theory claim you can avoid the negative consequences of lectins and thereby enjoy a happier, healthier life: You'll maintain your ideal weight, elevate your energy levels, and stave off the aging process.

But there is a complete absence of peer-reviewed documentation that supports the blood type diet, and the theories it is based on are flawed.

Consider the assertion that, when a person with type A blood eats meats or other high-protein sources, the lectins in these foods cause erythrocytes (red blood cells) to agglutinate (clump together). If true, this would have serious ramifications. Over time, the clumps of erythrocytes would become extremely large and clog up the body's vast network of capillaries (tiny blood vessels). This would impede blood flow and thereby prevent oxygen from being delivered to bodily tissues. Without a steady supply of oxygen, the vital organs would become irreparably damaged and, in short order, result in death. Not a pretty picture.

But while this scenario certainly sounds ominous, there is nothing to show that it actually occurs in real life. The scientific literature fails to reveal even one instance where food-induced agglutination of erythrocytes produced cardiovascular complications. If blood type really had such an effect on food, it would be common knowledge throughout the medical community. Sophisticated medical tests such as Doppler ultrasonography would clearly show the dire consequences from agglutinated red blood cells in those afflicted. Yet none of this data exists.

The blood type theory also states that, in addition to diet, blood type actually has an impact on your activity levels. Since type O's were hunters, they should engage in vigorous exercise; type A's, on the other hand, were docile agriculturalists and thus should engage in only gentle mind/body exercise. Yet there is nothing to show that people with type A blood have a decreased exercise response. Given the fact that moderate to intense exercise has clearly been shown to have a positive influence on body composition and longevity for all demographic groups,[4,5] it is highly counterproductive for *anyone* who is physically able to avoid intense training.

Even the anthropologic basis of blood types is highly questionable. It has not been scientifically established that type O was the original blood type. Blood typing didn't come about until 1901, when Austrian immunologist Karl Landsteiner identified the primary antigens and developed the accepted system of classification. Hence, it's a huge leap to assume that blood types evolved due to dietary concerns. Quite to the contrary, evidence seems to suggest that the ABO blood groups have been around since the dawn of humankind.[6] In fact, the AB type (which proponents of the diet say is the most recent blood group) apparently has a lineage that dates back more than 13 million years.[7]

While there are those who claim to have achieved remarkable success by following the blood type diet, any benefits are likely accidental. For instance, approximately 10 percent of the population are lactose intolerant.[8] Hence, there is a statistical probability that if a group of people with type O blood limited their consumption of dairy products, some of them would benefit from the action. But this in no way indicates that there's a cause-effect relationship between type O blood and restricting dairy products. It's simply a reflection of the elements of chance; if enough people follow a given diet, some are bound to experience positive results.

MYTH: You should perform cardiovascular exercise first thing in the morning on an empty stomach.

In an effort to burn more fat, it has become common practice for people to perform cardio as soon as they roll out of bed. Here's the philosophy: A prolonged absence of food brings about a reduction in circulating blood sugar, causing glycogen (stored carbohydrate) levels to fall. With a diminished availability of glycogen, your body tends to rely more on fat—rather than on glucose—to fuel your workout. Under ideal conditions, there is an increased oxidation of fat during exercise.[9] But although this might sound good in theory, it really doesn't apply in practice.

The human body is a very dynamic organism and continually adjusts its use of fat for fuel. This process is governed by a host of factors (including enzyme levels, substrate availability, internal feedback loops, etc.) that can literally change by the moment. Thus, simply looking at the amount of fat burned during exercise is shortsighted. Fat burning must be considered over the course of an entire day—not on an hour-to-hour basis—to have any meaning.

What's more, only about half of the fat utilized during aerobic exercise is mobilized from adipose tissue; the balance comes from fat stored intramuscularly (within muscle).[10] The important point here is that intramuscular fat has no bearing on aesthetic appearance; it's the subcutaneous fat stored in adipose tissue that influences body composition. Consequently, the actual fat-burning effects of the strategy are far less than it would appear.

In addition, studies have shown that eating before exercise actually increases caloric expenditure.[11] This apparently is related to the thermic effect of food (TEF).[12] As previously discussed, every time you eat a mixed meal, there is a corresponding increase in metabolic rate. When exercise is performed after the consumption of food, metabolism is heightened by about 20 percent over fasting levels. Better yet, these effects are maintained for up to three hours post-workout.[13]

Perhaps more significantly, a pre-exercise meal allows you to exercise more intensely.[14] In order to perform at a high level, your body needs a ready source of glycogen; deplete glycogen stores and your performance is bound to suffer. Compounding matters, not everyone functions well first thing in the morning. If you're more of a night owl, chances are that you'll sleepwalk through a morning workout. The net result is that fewer calories are burned during activity. Again, total caloric expenditure has a direct effect on fat oxidation, so these factors ultimately lead to a lower-quality, less-efficient exercise session.

All things considered, simply increasing the percentage of calories burned from fat doesn't translate into an improved body composition. There isn't necessarily anything wrong with performing exercise after an overnight fast, but it isn't going to make a significant difference in the appearance of your physique, either. The best advice is to exercise when you are at your best; let your biorhythms determine when you should work out. If you are a morning person, go ahead and train early. But if you don't really get going until you've been awake for several hours, by all means train later in the day. Either way, it's not going to make much of a difference in your results.

MYTH: It's beneficial to take supplemental free-form amino acids.

A popular strategy among athletes is to consume amino acids in their free form (as individual amino acids rather than as whole proteins). Branched chain amino acids (BCAAs), in particular, are favorites of bodybuilders and other strength athletes. Unlike most amino acids, which are metabolized by the liver, BCAAs are primarily taken up by the skeletal muscles and utilized for muscular function. So if you take extra BCAAs, it should theoretically improve your muscle development.

Unfortunately, taking BCAAs, or any other amino acids in their free form, doesn't work as advertised.[15] On the contrary, it is actually inferior to consuming whole proteins or protein peptides. In order to understand why, let's revisit how proteins are digested. The absorption of amino acids begins in the small intestine, where they must pass through the intestinal brush border before being taken up by intestinal cells. The process, however, requires an active carrier system. As the name implies, this system actively transports amino acids across the intestinal brush border for assimilation.

Here's the kicker, though. In their free-form state, amino acids use the same carrier system and therefore compete with one another for entry. When a particular amino acid is consumed in abundance, it can impair absorption of other amino acids, leading to an imbalance. This can cause the breakdown of internal proteins, especially those in your muscles, to replenish the body's supply of the deficient amino acids—not a desirable scenario.

The human body is actually more adept at digesting amino acids as peptides (which are obtained from the digestion of whole foods or specially formulated supplements). Peptides have their own carrier systems that provide transport across the intestinal brush border.[16] The difference, though, is that the peptide carrier system has a larger transport capacity than the carrier system for single amino acids, promoting better absorption, and therefore better growth, than free-form amino acids.[17]

So forget about taking free-form amino acids. It is not only superfluous, but potentially counterproductive. At best, all you'll get is expensive urine; at worst, you can impair nutrient absorption and cause an amino acid imbalance. Provided you take in adequate dietary protein (approximately one gram of protein per pound of body weight), you'll get a full complement of essential and nonessential amino acids, including all the BCAAs that you need.

MYTH: You can get rid of a "problem area" by performing specific exercises.

Picture this scenario: It's late at night and you're watching television. While changing channels, you see a fitness show that grabs your interest. A muscular guy with six-pack abs is hawking a device called the Ab Buster on a set that's glitzier than a Las Vegas variety show. Soon thereafter, he is joined by a bevy of sexy fitness models who ogle at his extraordinary abdominal development, making it clear that a flat, toned midsection is the best way to a woman's heart. "If you buy this unit today," he proclaims, "you can lose two inches off your waist by next month. And it's so easy to use, you barely have to exert any effort to get results."

Despite these lofty claims, there's no way to spot-reduce body fat; it's a physiologic impossibility. Individual exercises can't slim down a specific area of your body—no matter how often or intensely you perform the movement.[18] All the sit-ups in the world won't give you a flat stomach; no amount of lower-body exercises will directly diminish the size of your thighs. In reality, trying to eradicate your problem areas with targeted movements is literally an exercise in futility.

In order to appreciate why spot reduction doesn't work, it is necessary to review a little biochemistry. When calories are consumed in abundance, your body converts the excess nutrients into fat-based compounds called *triglycerides,* which are then stored in adipocytes (fat cells). If you remember, adipocytes are pliable storehouses that either shrink or expand to accommodate fatty deposits.

When you exercise, triglycerides are broken back down into fatty acids, which are then transported via the blood to be used in target tissues for energy.[19] Because fatty acids must travel through the bloodstream—a time-consuming event—it is just as efficient for your body to utilize fat from one area as it is another. In other words, the proximity of fat cells to the working muscles is completely irrelevant from an energy standpoint. Since the body can't preferentially use fat from a particular area, it draws from adipocytes in all regions of the body, including the face, trunk, and extremities. It's that simple.

Fortunately, all is not lost in the battle of the bulge. By following the protocol laid out in this book, you will get lean, even in those hard-to-lose areas. Just give it some time and you will see results—guaranteed!

MYTH: If you stop lifting weights, your muscle will turn to fat.

It's pretty much common knowledge that intense exercise improves muscular development. But what happens if you stop working out? There is a prevailing sentiment that, when training is ceased, the process reverses and all the muscle that you've acquired just turns into fat. This belief is often an argument against strength training. After all, why go to all the trouble of building your muscles if they're just going to morph into adipose once training is discontinued.

The truth is, however, muscle and fat are two separate and distinct properties that have completely different molecular structures. Muscle is a protein-based tissue composed of filaments called actin and myosin. Body fat, on the other hand, consists of stored triglycerides, which are made up of a carbohydrate (glycerol) and three fatty acids. Hence, the possibility of muscle turning into fat (or vice versa) is akin to an apple becoming an orange: There's simply no mechanism for it to happen.

"But what about retired athletes?" I'm often asked. It's all too common to see former football or baseball players whose once buff bodies are now soft and flabby. How do you explain this seeming transformation from muscle to fat?

The answer can be traced to caloric balance: the amount of calories expended versus consumed. You see, athletes tend to become sedentary once their competitive careers are over.[20] They no longer participate in the intense games and practice sessions—activities that burn up more than 1,000 calories at a pop. To make matters worse, they often abandon their strength-training programs, causing muscle tissue to atrophy (get smaller). If you remember, muscle is highly metabolically active—it burns a substantial amount of calories, even at rest. As muscular density diminishes, there is a corresponding decrease in metabolic rate. The net effect of this double whammy: caloric expenditure is significantly lower than it was during their professional careers.

The problem is that these same athletes often don't adjust their caloric intake after retirement. They'll continue to scoff down mass quantities of food without regard to their activity levels. Consequently, energy balance becomes skewed in favor of a caloric surplus, inevitably causing an increase in body fat. And with less muscle and more adipose tissue, there is the illusion that muscle has turned into fat.

The good news is that it really doesn't require a significant time commitment to preserve muscular gains. In fact, you need only work out a few times a month to keep yourself in good shape! Studies have shown that a single training session every ten to fourteen days is all that's necessary to prevent the breakdown of muscle tissue.[21] Only during long periods of complete inactivity does muscular atrophy set in. As long as you don't completely abstain from training, metabolism remains elevated, making it easier to maintain a lean physique.

So don't let the "muscle-to-fat myth" deter you from lifting weights. The only thing that happens when you stop training is that your muscles begin to atrophy, eventually returning to pre-exercise levels. To avoid unwanted weight gain, you must obey the laws of thermodynamics and match caloric intake to caloric expenditure. When an exercise program is discontinued, you need to reassess your eating habits and take in fewer calories to account for a slower metabolism and reduced activity levels. If calories are not reduced, you'll ultimately gain weight and give the illusion of having your muscle turn into fat.

MYTH: To burn fat, it's better to do low-intensity aerobic activities than high-intensity activities.

Distressingly, some fitness professionals have perpetrated the myth that, for optimal fat burning, aerobics should be performed at a low level of intensity. For example, they advocate walking, instead of running, as a means to shift the body into a "fat-burning zone." This theory is predicated on the fact that a greater proportion of fat is burned during low-intensity exercise as opposed to exercise done at a higher level of intensity.[22]

The truth is, however, that the selective use of fat for fuel doesn't necessarily translate into a greater amount of fat loss. Consider that, during complete rest, almost 90 percent of energy expenditure is derived from fat stores. If the percentage of fat calories were the overriding factor in fat loss, then watching TV would make you skinny!

In reality, the loss of body fat is contingent on the total amount of fat calories burned—not the percentage of calories derived from fat—and, from this standpoint, high-intensity exercise invariably comes out ahead. For example, if you burn 200 calories in a half hour by walking on the treadmill at a low level of intensity, approximately 60 percent of these calories will come from fat, giving you a net fat loss of 120 calories. On the other hand, exercising for the same amount of time at a high intensity will burn approximately 400 calories with 160 of these calories coming from fat (even though the percentage of calories derived from fat is only 40 percent). So while it's true that the *ratio* of fat burned is greater with low-intensity activities, exercising at higher intensities burns more fat on an absolute basis.[23]

High-intensity cardio also has a positive effect on weight loss immediately following exercise.[24] After finishing a training session, there is fair amount of excess postexercise oxygen consumption (EPOC); your metabolism remains elevated for a protracted period of time. But only high-intensity exercise has a profound impact on EPOC. It burns about twice as many calories as a comparable low-intensity activity with results lasting for up to several hours post-workout.[25] All told, there is both a greater total amount of calories expended as well as a greater amount of fat oxidation.[26]

Further, when you consider the time-related efficiency of training, low-intensity exercise provides a very poor cost/benefit dividend. Nothing is more laborious than walking on a treadmill for protracted periods. Why would you want to spend an hour exercising when you can get similar results from training for half that time?

So it is misguided to believe that low-intensity aerobics are best for burning fat. There is a direct correlation between physical effort and caloric expenditure; the harder you work, the more calories you expend. Accordingly, high-intensity exercise burns more fat calories on an absolute basis than low-intensity activities. And since the most important aspect of weight loss is the total amount of fat calories burned—not the percentage from fat—training should be performed at the highest intensity possible. Thus, if fat burning is your aim, performing cardiovascular exercise at a high level of intensity is clearly your best bet.

MYTH: You shouldn't exercise during pregnancy.

Sadly, a majority of women still believe that pregnancy requires a sedentary lifestyle. They adhere to the old-school attitude that exercise can somehow harm the fetus. Even many gynecologists are uninformed about the subject and continue to counsel their patients to avoid any type of strenuous physical activity.

The truth is, virtually every woman can and should stay active throughout pregnancy. When properly implemented, an exercise regimen can provide a multitude of benefits for the pregnant woman, with virtually no downside.

During pregnancy, a woman undergoes many physiologic and hormonal changes that can alter her metabolism and body shape. It is commonplace to gain thirty, forty, or even fifty pounds postpartum, and most women are unprepared to deal with this event. But while it is certainly possible to get back into shape after pregnancy, the best way to counteract postpartum weight gain is to stay in shape *during* pregnancy. By remaining dedicated to a workout schedule, a woman can virtually return to her original shape shortly after delivery.

Moreover, adopting a workout routine helps to increase energy levels and reduce the fatigue associated with pregnancy. It is common for a woman to sit around the house all day, feeling unattractive and lethargic as her term progresses. Some are so self-conscious about their appearance that they avoid social situations altogether. By promoting a better sense of well-being, exercise helps to improve self-esteem during this fragile period.

Numerous other exercise-related benefits have been reported, including a lower incidence of back pain, reduced edema, and fewer leg cramps.[27] What's more, there is a positive influence on delivery. Research demonstrates that women who train during pregnancy experience a shorter active labor and a decreased amount of fetal stress.[28] It has even been shown that the offspring of women who exercise have significantly lower body-fat levels than those who remain sedentary—even after a five-year follow-up period![29]

There are, though, many unique principles to pregnancy training, and extensive care must be taken to ensure a safe, effective workout. The goal of exercise during pregnancy should be to maintain the highest level of fitness consistent with maximum safety. By understanding the basic guidelines of pregnancy training and adopting a dedicated workout program, a woman can reap all the rewards of staying fit during and after pregnancy without risking injury to herself or to her fetus. For further information, consult my book *Sculpting Her Body Perfect,* which has an entire chapter on the subject.

MYTH: You can get rid of cellulite by using herbal remedies.

How many times have you seen ads for "magic potions" that claim to "melt away" cellulite? Dating back to the nineteenth century, charlatans have made a fortune by hawking these "miracle" products. Creams, lotions, ointments . . . just rub them on and watch your dimpled skin disappear. Sound too good to be true? Well, it is.

Cellulite is a genetic condition that can't be purged by magic potions.[30] You see, cellulite tends to be hereditary; if your mother and siblings are afflicted, the chances are good that you will be too. Like your height, eye color, and hair texture, genetics dictate where fat is deposited and the semblance that it takes on your body. Hence, while some women can be obese with little evidence of cellulite, others can be relatively thin and have cottage cheese thighs. This is simply the luck of the draw. If you picked good parents, you might escape the big "C." If not . . .

Interestingly, men rarely develop cellulite. This is due to the composition of human skin. The skin and its underlying tissue have three fundamental layers: The top layer is made up of a cellular-based tissue called the dermis. Its primary purpose is to protect your body from outside contaminants. The middle layer is made up of fibrous connective tissue called superficial fascia. It is substantially thicker than the dermis and acts like an internal stocking to support the skin. The lower layer is made up of adipose tissue—plain old fat. It has several functions including insulating the body, padding the internal organs, and providing a source of long-term energy.

You're probably wondering how all this physiology applies to cellulite. Well, the superficial fascia is responsible for holding body fat in place. In men, the superficial fascia is arranged in a crisscross pattern that is strong and consistent. Accordingly, fat is contained in a uniform manner subcutaneously (below the skin), leaving the skin surface smooth and supple. In women, however, the superficial fascia tends to be irregular and discontinuous.[31] It has a vertical distribution, forming honeycomb-like patterns beneath the dermis. Hence, when fat accumulates, it pushes up toward the skin's surface in clusters, giving the skin the lumpy, dimpled appearance commonly known as cellulite.

Cellulite is further exacerbated by the localized accumulation of lymphatic fluid. Research has shown that cellulite contains an abundance of glycosaminoglycans—a polysaccharide-based compound that has high water-attracting properties.[32] Glycosaminoglycans draw fluid into fatty tissue, causing extensive swelling in cellulite-affected areas.

Given that cellulite is related to the structural composition of connective tissue, it's easy to see why it's impossible for a cream to eradicate the problem; there's simply no way for an externally applied solution to penetrate the skin and "reconfigure" the underlying connective tissue. For all intents and purposes, anything short of radical surgery simply has no lasting effect on the condition.[33]

But just because you may be predisposed to cellulite doesn't mean you have to succumb to its effects. A combination of proper nutrition and regimented exercise is the only viable way to counteract the problem. By reducing body fat and adding muscle tone, you can substantially reduce, if not completely eliminate, this unsightly malady. Muscle helps to smooth underlying fat, making dimples less evident. And once body fat is reduced to acceptable levels, cellulite-prone areas will appear taut and toned rather than lumpy and bumpy.

MYTH: Liposuction is a permanent answer to fat loss.

Liposuction (lipo, for short) is perhaps the most controversial weight-loss option. In just a few short years, it has become one of the most commonly performed elective surgeries in the world. Doctors market the procedure as a way to "contour" the body. Just suck out the fat, they assert, and you'll never again have to worry about being overweight. But despite this lofty proclamation, it's really not that cut and dried.

Liposuction is a medical procedure performed by a licensed physician. A cylindrical tube is inserted into a fatty area and fat is literally "vacuumed" from the body. It usually is done under local anesthesia on an outpatient basis, making it relatively convenient and safe (although several deaths have been attributed to the procedure).

For the most part, lipo is reasonably effective at removing small amounts of localized fat. The technique has been perfected to the point where there isn't much scarring or discomfort. Recovery is fairly short, and, although swelling temporarily obscures results, visible changes can be seen almost immediately.

The trouble is, the effects of liposuction aren't permanent. Regardless of what some cosmetic surgeons would have you believe, without proper exercise and nutrition, body fat will return. Excess calories have to be stored somewhere and, rest assured, they'll find their way into fat cells. Areas of the body that never stored much fat will begin to enlarge. The arms, back, neck—places you normally don't associate with fat storage suddenly start to appear pudgy.

And don't think treated areas are immune from regaining weight. Lipo only removes a small percentage of fat cells from a site. There are plenty of existing adipocytes left that are hungry for fat. Once these cells reach a certain size, they undergo a process called hyperplasia, where they divide into more fat cells.[34,35] That's right, fat cells can regenerate! I've consulted with many women who've gone through the travails and expense of lipo only to wind up right back where they started.

So if you're considering lipo, do it with the proper perspective. While it's possible to remove small pockets of fat from select places, you must follow it up with regimented diet and exercise. If not, you're just wasting your time and money.

MYTH: Consuming high amounts of protein causes osteoporosis.

One of the biggest arguments against consuming a diet high in protein is that it can lead to osteoporosis. Here's the rationale: The digestion of protein causes an increase in stomach acids—much more so than the other macronutrients. In response, the body starts breaking down bone minerals, which act as an acid buffer, to neutralize pH. Conceivably, a large protein intake can cause excessive calcium loss and, ultimately, loss of bone tissue.

It has been shown, however, that as long as an adequate amount of dietary calcium is consumed, excess protein intake has little effect on bone health.[36] This is significant since protein-rich foods generally contain high levels of calcium; as protein consumption increases, so does calcium.[37] Thus, any negative effects of a high protein diet tend to be counterbalanced by greater calcium intake.

In support of this fact, consider the eating habits of cavemen, who subsisted largely on meat, poultry, and fish. Given their reliance on dietary protein, you might predict that cavemen would have shown premature signs of osteoporosis. Yet fossil records show quite the opposite to be true. Stone Age humans actually had thick bones with large cortical cross-sectional areas, much denser than that of contemporary humans.[38] Why? Their calcium intake was more than double that in today's society![39]

Similar results are seen in today's population. Not only is there a lack of evidence that protein intake is associated with bone loss, studies show a positive correlation with mineral density in the legs, arms, and spine.[40,41,42] Given the facts, there is reason to believe that consuming more protein can actually help to stave off osteoporosis and reduce the risk of debilitating fractures![43]

So don't fret about eating a higher-protein diet. Provided you consume a variety of protein-rich foods, you'll go a long way to ensuring adequate calcium intake (approximately 1,000 to 1,500 milligrams a day). In addition, make sure to include ample amounts of fruits and vegetables. These foods act as alkaline buffers and therefore aid in the preservation of skeletal calcium stores.[44] And finally, when in doubt take a multivitamin/mineral complex that contains calcium. This serves as an insurance policy, protecting against a possible deficiency.

CHAPTER 15

Look Great Naked Recipes

You really can eat healthy foods that actually taste great! Just because a dish is low in saturated fat and sugar doesn't mean that it has to be bland.

I asked some of the top fitness models and bodybuilders in the world—people who make their living by looking great—to submit their favorite healthy recipes and, on the pages that follow, are their mouth-watering responses. You'll find everything from breakfast, lunch, and dinner entrées, to delicious snacks. And best of all, most of the recipes take only minutes to prepare!

So go ahead and indulge yourself. Eat like a champion and enjoy!

DEEANN'S CHICKEN IN MUSTARD SAUCE

DeeAnn Donovan
Mrs. New York International
www.DeeAnnModel.com

- 4 chicken breast halves, boned and skinned
- 1 tablespoon olive oil
- 1 cup apple juice
- 1 medium onion, peeled and sliced very thin
- 1 garlic clove, peeled and minced
- 1½ teaspoons fresh thyme leaves
- 2 tablespoons Dijon mustard
- 1 apple, cored and sliced

Place the chicken breast halves between two sheets of waxed paper. With the broad side of a heavy knife, pound the chicken breasts to flatten them to about ½ inch thick. Heat the oil in a large skillet over medium-high heat until hot. Add the chicken and sauté for about 3 minutes on each side or until golden. Add the apple juice, onion, garlic, and thyme. Cover and cook for 10 minutes or until the chicken is fork-tender. Remove the chicken and keep it warm. Heat the liquid remaining in the skillet to boiling. Blend in the mustard. Add the apple slices and cook until heated through. Pour the sauce over the chicken and enjoy!

BETHANY'S BEEF TACO SALAD

Bethany Carter Howlett, M.S., CSCS
IFBB Fitness Professional
Better Bodies By Bethany, Inc.
www.bethanyhowlett.com

- 1 pound extra-lean ground beef
- 1 onion, chopped
- 1 package taco seasoning mix (or season meat with chili powder)
- 1 cup pinto or black beans, rinsed and drained
- 1 pinch chopped fresh cilantro

- 4 cups shredded lettuce
- 6 ounces shredded fat-free cheddar cheese
- 2 tomatoes, chopped
- Bunch of fresh cilantro, washed and chopped
- 6 tablespoons light sour cream
- 1 green onion, chopped
- Salsa of your choice

In a large nonstick skillet, brown ground beef with onion. Cook until well done, not pink. Drain off fat and add taco mix with water per package directions, along with beans and a sprinkle of cilantro. Continue cooking according to package directions or until the ingredients are thoroughly combined. Arrange six individual salad plates starting with a small layer of shredded lettuce, then top with beef/bean mixture, shredded cheese, tomatoes, and cilantro. In the center, add 1 tablespoon sour cream, sprinkle with chopped green onion, and add a dollop of salsa. Depending on how many days you went to the gym this week, you can start with a layer of baked chips on the bottom. As a colorful garnish, stick a red or green corn chip in the center and enjoy!

AMANDA'S MEXICAN FIESTA LOAF

Amanda Doerrer
IFBB Fitness Professional
www.amandadoerrer.com

- 1 pound extra-lean ground turkey
- ½ cup dry oats
- 2 egg whites
- ¼ cup fresh salsa
- 2 tablespoons hot sauce (or to taste)
- 1 teaspoon black pepper (or to taste)
- ½ large onion, chopped
- ⅓ cup black pinto beans, drained
- ¼ cup shredded low-fat cheddar cheese

Preheat oven to 375°F. In a bowl, combine turkey, oats, and egg whites. Stir in the salsa, hot sauce, black pepper, and onion. Add the pinto beans and cheese. Stir until just mixed. Spoon into a loaf pan and bake for one hour and enjoy!

KRISTIA'S OATMEAL PROTEIN PANCAKES

Kristia Knowles
IFBB Fitness Professional
www.kristiaknowles.net

- 2 cups slow-cooking oatmeal
- 12 egg whites
- 2 scoops flavored protein powder (12 grams of protein per scoop)
- 1 ounce of almonds

Preheat skillet to 350°F. Mix all of the ingredients together in a bowl. Pour generous portions of the batter onto the skillet. Cook pancakes until lightly brown on both sides and enjoy!

RICH'S TUNA SURPRISE

Rich Gaspari
IFBB Professional Bodybuilder
Arnold Classic Champion
www.richgaspari.com

- 5 egg whites
- 1 can of solid white albacore tuna, liquid drained
- ¼ cup grated Parmesan cheese
- 3 garlic cloves, crushed
- ½ onion, sliced
- 1 cup cooked brown rice

In a bowl, mix together egg whites, tuna, and cheese. Spray a nonstick pan with nonstick cooking spray and sauté crushed garlic and sliced onions over medium heat until transparent. Pour tuna mixture over onions and garlic and cook over low heat until egg whites are no longer transparent. Serve over brown rice and enjoy!

LAURA'S CHEESEBURGER PIE

Laura Mak
IFBB Fitness Professional
www.lauramak.com

- 1 pound lean ground turkey or lean ground beef
- ¼ cup chopped green pepper
- ¼ cup chopped onion
- 1 tomato, sliced
- 1 cup vegetarian spaghetti sauce
- ½ cup low-fat cheddar cheese
- ½ cup low-fat mozzarella cheese

Preheat oven to 350°F. Spread a half-inch layer of meat on the bottom of a round glass pie pan. Bake for about 10 minutes or until it looks medium well. Remove from the oven and drain the juices. Add green pepper, onion, and tomato. Spread sauce on the top, covering the veggies. Sprinkle cheeses over the sauce. Bake for another 5 minutes or until the cheese has melted. Allow a few minutes to cool before you slice and enjoy!

JULIE'S FAT-FREE LEMON CHEESECAKE

Julie Palmer
IFBB Fitness Professional
www.juliepalmer.com

- 1 cup water
- 1 packet sugar-free lemon Jell-O
- 16 ounces fat-free cream cheese
- 12 ounces fat-free Cool Whip
- 1 fat-free pie crust

Boil water and stir in Jell-O until dissolved. Turn off heat and let cool slightly. Once cooled but not gelled, mix cream cheese and Cool Whip into the mixture and stir well. Pour the contents into the pie crust, chill in the refrigerator overnight, and enjoy!

STELLA'S EASY BEEF AND BROCCOLI

Stella Juarez
Author: Stella's Kitchen
www.bodybuilding.about.com
www.stellaskitchen.com

- 2 teaspoons minced garlic (about 6 cloves)
- ¼ cup reduced-sodium beef broth
- 1 pound top round or flank steak (cut in strips or small pieces)
- 4 cups chopped broccoli (about 2 medium heads)
- ½ medium yellow onion, roughly chopped
- Fresh ground pepper, to taste

Preheat wok or skillet and sauté garlic in ½ tablespoon of the broth for 1 minute. Add beef and cook until meat has almost reached your desired level of doneness. Add broccoli, onions, the remaining beef broth, and pepper, and cook until vegetables have softened. Covering the pan with a lid for a few minutes will accelerate the cooking time of this last step. Serve over brown rice and enjoy!

NICOLE'S SALMON SUPREME

Nicole Caballer
Team Universe Champion
Email: Nicnacfitness@aol.com

- 3 tablespoons olive oil
- 1 whole egg
- 5 egg whites
- 1 pound salmon fillets
- 1 cup dry oats, finely chopped
- Mrs. Dash Garlic & Herb seasoning to taste

Heat olive oil in a skillet over medium heat. Whisk whole egg and egg whites in a bowl. Dip each salmon fillet in egg, then coat with oats. Add salmon fillets to skillet. Sprinkle Mrs. Dash over salmon, and cook for 4 to 6 minutes (until oats brown). Flip salmon over, sprinkle with Mrs. Dash, and cook for another 4 minutes or so, and enjoy!

LAURA'S BREAKFAST FAJITA

Laura Creavalle
IFBB Ms. International
www.lauracreavalle.com

- 5 egg whites (or about one cup fat-free egg substitute)
- 1 tablespoon chopped green onion
- 1 ounce fat-free cheddar cheese
- 2 fat-free whole-wheat flour tortillas
- 2 tablespoons salsa
- 1 tablespoon fat-free sour cream (optional)

Whisk together egg whites and pour into a nonstick skillet sprayed with cooking spray. Add green onion and cook over medium heat. Turn eggs over once, sprinkle with cheese, cover skillet, and remove from heat. Warm tortillas in a microwave oven for 20 seconds. Place egg in tortilla and roll up. Add salsa and sour cream and enjoy!

Orexins and Anorexins

Orexins	Anorexins
Neuropeptide Y (NPY)	Corticotropin-releasing hormone (CRH)
Melanin-concentrating hormone (MCH)	Cholecystokinin (CCK)
Galanin	Cocaine-and-amphetamine-regulated transcript (CART)
Beta-endorphin	Melanocyte-stimulating hormone (MSH)
Dynorphin	GLP-1
Agouti-related protein (AGRP)	Bombesin
Growth hormone–releasing hormone (GHRH)	Serotonin
Ghrelin	Somatostatin
	Thyrotropin-releasing hormone (TRH)
	Peptide YY189 (PYY)

Resources

USDA Nutrient Values: www.rahul.net/cgi-bin/fatfree/usda/usda.cgi   *A searchable database for the nutrient values of many different foods.*

ConsumerLab: www.consumerlab.com.   *This site evaluates the quality of various supplements. Products that pass their testing protocol get the ConsumerLab Seal of Approval.*

Supplement Watch: www.supplementwatch.com   *An excellent compilation of reviews on various herbs and other supplements.*

FDA/CFSAN Web site: www.cfsan.fda.gov/~dms/ds-savvy.html   *This site is titled "Tips for the Savvy Supplement User: Making Informed Decisions and Evaluating Information" and contains some good advice about dietary supplementation.*

Look Great Naked Web site: www.lookgreatnaked.com   *My own site, containing a vast array of information and resources on a variety of fitness topics.*

NUTRITION BOOKS

Advanced Nutrition and Human Metabolism by James L. Groff and Sareen S. Gropper (Wadsworth Publishing, 1999). *One of the best all-around nutrition texts available. A good background in science is necessary to grasp much of the information.*

Biochemical and Physiological Aspects of Human Nutrition by Martha H. Stipanuk (W. B. Saunders, 2000). *The most complete book on all aspects of nutrition that I have ever read. Be forewarned, though: An extensive background in science is required.*

Fats That Heal, Fats That Kill by Udo Erasmus (Alive Books, 1993). *A nice overview on how different types of fats affect your body and health.*

The Complete Book of Food Counts by Corinne T. Netzer (Dell Publishing, 2000). *A listing of just about every food you can think of with corresponding values for protein, fat, carbohydrate, cholesterol, fiber, and sodium. Good for getting a handle on your portions.*

Stella's Kitchen by Stella C. Juarez (On Target Publications, 2003). *A wide-ranging collection of tasty, healthy recipes that are sure to satisfy everyone's taste buds.*

EXERCISE BOOKS

Sculpting Her Body Perfect by Brad Schoenfeld (Human Kinetics, 2002). *A comprehensive training program for women looking to maximize their bodies' potential, with routines from beginner to advanced levels.*

Look Great at Any Age by Brad Schoenfeld (Prentice Hall Press, 2003). *A streamlined, time-efficient program for women looking to get into shape. Aimed at those aged thirty-five and over but can be effective for all ages.*

Strength Training Anatomy by Frédéric Delavier (Human Kinetics, 2001). *Well-detailed anatomical drawings of all the major muscle groups and how they are involved in various exercises.*

Designing Resistance Training Programs by Steven J. Fleck and William J. Kraemer (Human Kinetics, 1997). *Good primer on exercise basics and how to customize a program to various needs and goals.*

Supertraining by Mel Siff (Supertraining Institute, 2000) *Perhaps the most comprehensive book on exercise ever written. The author is one of the most brilliant minds in the field. Highly recommended.*

Notes

CHAPTER 1

1. Mokdad AH, et al. The continuing epidemics of obesity and diabetes in the United States. *JAMA*, 2001 Sep 12;286(10):1195–200.

2. Sturm R, et al. Does obesity contribute as much to morbidity as poverty or smoking? *Public Health*, 2001 May;115(3):229–35.

3. Blendon RJ, et al. Americans' views on the use and regulation of dietary supplements. *Arch Intern Med*, 2001 Mar 26;161(6):805–10.

4. Flegal KM, et al. Prevalence and Trends in Obesity Among US Adults, 1999–2000. *JAMA*, 2002;288:1723–27.

5. Arner P. Control of lipolysis and its relevance to development of obesity in man. *Diabetes Metab Rev*, 1988 Aug;4(5):507–15. Review.

6. Lafontan M, et al. Fat cell alpha 2-adrenoceptors: the regulation of fat cell function and lipolysis. *Endocr Rev*, 1995 Dec;16(6):716–38. Review.

7. Herrera E, et al. Lipid metabolism in the fetus and the newborn. *Diabetes Metab Res Rev*, 2000 May–Jun;16(3):202–10. Review.

8. Pratley R, et al. Strength training increases resting metabolic rate and norepinephrine levels in healthy 50- to 65-yr-old men. *J Appl Physiol*, 1994 Jan;76(1): 133–7.

9. Robergs RA, et al. *Exercise Physiology: Exercise, Performance and Clinical Applications*. Boston: WCB McGraw-Hill, 1997.

10. Kissebah AH, et al. Relation of body fat distribution to metabolic complications of obesity. *J Clin Endocrinol Metab*, 1982 Feb;54(2):254–60.

11. Wahrenberg H, et al. Mechanisms underlying regional differences in lipolysis in human adipose tissue. *J Clin Invest*, 1989 Aug;84(2):458–67.

12. Blaak E. Gender differences in fat metabolism. *Curr Opin Clin Nutr Metab Care*, 2001 Nov;4(6):499–502. Review.

13. Rebuffe-Scrive M, et al. Regional adipose tissue metabolism in men and post-menopausal women. *Int J Obes*, 1987;11(4):347–55.

14. Rebuffe-Scrive M, et al. Metabolism of mammary, abdominal, and femoral adipocytes in women before and after menopause. *Metabolism*, 1986 Sep;35(9):792–7.

15. Björntorp P. The regulation of adipose tissue distribution in humans. *Int J Obes Relat Metab Disord*, 1996 Apr;20(4):291–302.

16. Roncari DA. Hormonal influences on the replication and maturation of adipocyte precursors. *Int J Obes*, 1981;5(6):547–52.

17. Schwartz SM, et al. Effects of estradiol and progesterone on food intake, body weight, and carcass adiposity in weanling rats. *Am J Physiol*, 1981 May;240(5): E499–503.

18. Wajchenberg BL. Subcutaneous and visceral adipose tissue: Their relation to the metabolic syndrome. *Endocr Rev*, 2000 Dec;21(6):697–738. Review.

19. Berman DM, et al. Regional differences in adrenoceptor binding and fat cell lipolysis in obese, postmenopausal women. *Metabolism*, 1998 Apr;47(4):467–73.

20. Stunkard AJ, et al. An adoption study of human obesity. *N Engl J Med*, 1986 Jan 23;314(4):193–8.

21. Bouchard C, et al. Heredity and body fat. *Annu Rev Nutr*, 1988;8:259–77. Review.

22. Sorenson TI, et al. Childhood body mass index—genetic and familial environmental influences assessed in a longitudinal adoption study. *Int J Obes Relat Metab Disord*, 1992 Sep;16(9):705–14.

23. Stunkard AJ, et al. The body-mass index of twins who have been reared apart. *N Engl J Med*, 1990 May 24;322(21):1483–7.

24. Lev-Ran A. Human obesity: An evolutionary approach to understanding our bulging waistline. *Diabetes Metab Res Rev*, 2001 Sep–Oct;17(5):347–62. Review.

CHAPTER 2

1. Hetherington A, et al. Hypothalamic lesions and adiposity in the rat. *Anatomical Record*, 1940;78:149–72.

2. Kennedy GC. The role of depot fat in the hypothalamic control of food intake in the rat. *Proc R Soc Lond B Biol Sci*, 1953;140:579–92.

3. Zhang Y, et al. Positional cloning of the mouse obese gene and its human homologue. *Nature*, 1994 Dec 1;372(6505):425–32.

4. Banks WA, et al. Serum leptin levels in wild and captive populations of baboons (papio): Implications for the ancestral role of leptin. *J Clin Endocrinol Metab*, 2001 Sep;86(9):4315–20.

5. Maffei MJ, et al. Leptin levels in human and rodent: Measurement of plasma leptin and ob RNA in obese and weight-reduced subjects. *Nat Med*, 1995 Nov;1(11):1155–61.

6. Considine RV, et al. Evidence against either a premature stop codon or the absence of obese gene mRNA in human obesity. *J Clin Invest*, 1995 Jun;95(6): 2986–8.

7. Lonnqvist FP, et al. Leptin secretion from adipose tissue in women. Relationship to plasma levels and gene expression. *J Clin Invest*, 1997 May 15;99(10): 2398–404.

8. Rosenbaum M, et al. Leptin: A molecular integrating somatic energy stores energy expenditure and fertility. *Trends Endocrin Metab*, 1998;9:117–124.

9. Meier CA. Orexins and anorexins: Thoughts for food. *Eur J Endocrinol*, 1998 Aug;139(2):148–9. Review.

10. Rosenbaum M, et al. Effects of gender, body composition, and menopause on plasma concentrations of leptin. *J Clin Endocrin Metab*, 1996;81:3424–7.

11. Rosenbaum M, et al. A comparative study of different means of assessing long-term energy expenditure in humans. *Am J Physiol*, 1996;270:R496–R504.

12. Leibel R, et al. Changes in energy expenditure resulting from altered body weight. *New Engl J Med*, 1995;332:621–8.

13. Considine RV, et al. Serum immunoreactive-leptin concentrations in normal weight and obese humans. *New Engl J Med*, 1996;334:292–5.

14. Rosenbaum M, et al. Effect of weight change on plasma leptin concentrations and energy expenditure. *J Clin Endocrin Metab*, 1997;82:3647–54.

15. Banks WA, et al. Leptin enters the brain by a saturable system independent of insulin. *Peptides*, 1996;17(2):305–11.

16. Banks WA. Leptin transport across the blood-brain barrier: Implications for the cause and treatment of obesity. *Curr Pharm Des*, 2001 Jan;7(2):125–33. Review.

17. Lee JH, et al. Leptin resistance is associated with extreme obesity and aggregates in families. *Int J Obes Relat Metab Disord*, 2001 Oct;25(10):1471–3.

18. Wang J, et al. Overfeeding rapidly induces leptin and insulin resistance. *Diabetes*, 2001 Dec;50(12):2786–91.

19. Gabriely I, et al. Leptin resistance during aging is independent of fat mass. *Diabetes*, 2002 Apr;51(4):1016–21.

20. Lin L, et al. Acute changes in the response to peripheral leptin with alteration in the diet composition. *Am J Physiol Regul Integr Comp Physiol*, 2001 Feb;280(2):R504–9.

21. Air EL, et al. Insulin and leptin combine additively to reduce food intake and body weight in rats. *Endocrinology*, 2002 Jun;143(6):2449–52.

22. Campfield LA, et al. Transient declines in blood glucose signal meal initiation. *Int J Obes*, 1990;14 Suppl 3:15–31; discussion 31–4. Review.

23. Campfield LA, et al. On-line continuous measurement of blood glucose and meal pattern in free-feeding rats: The role of glucose in meal initiation. *Brain Res Bull*, 1985 Jun;14(6):605–16.

24. Louis-Sylvestre J, et al. Fall in blood glucose level precedes meal onset in free-feeding rats. *Neurosci Biobehav Rev*, 1980;4 Suppl 1:13–5.

25. Woods SC, et al. Insulin as an adiposity signal. *Int J Obes Relat Metab Disord*, 2001 Dec;25 Suppl 5:S35–8. Review.

26. Nakazato M, et al. A role for ghrelin in the central regulation of feeding. *Nature*, 2001 Jan 11;409(6817):194–8.

27. Witt KA, et al. Exercise training and dietary carbohydrate: Effects on selected hormones and the thermic effect of feeding. *Int J Sport Nutr*, 1993 Sep;3(3): 272–89.

28. De Jonge L, et al. The thermic effect of food and obesity: A critical review. *Obes Res*, 1997 Nov;5(6):622–31. Review.

29. Levin BE. Metabolic imprinting on genetically predisposed neural circuits perpetuates obesity. *Nutrition*, 2000 Oct;16(10):909–15. Review.

30. Levin BE. Diet cycling and age alter weight gain and insulin levels in rats. *Am J Physiol*, 1994 Aug;267(2 Pt 2):R527–35.

31. Keesey RE, et al. Body weight set-points: Determination and adjustment. *J Nutr*, 1997 Sep;127(9):1875S–83S. Review.

32. Vogler GP, et al. Influences of genes and shared family environment on adult body mass index assessed in an adoption study by a comprehensive path model. *Int J Obes Relat Metab Disord*, 1995 Jan;19(1):40–5.

33. Ravussin E, et al. Energy balance and weight regulation: Genetics versus environment. *Br J Nutr*, 2000 Mar;83 Suppl 1:S17–20. Review.

34. De Castro JM. What are the major correlates of macronutrient selection in Western populations? *Proc Nutr Soc*, 1999 Nov;58(4):755–63. Review.

35. Hill AJ. Developmental issues in attitudes to food and diet. *Proc Nutr Soc*, 2002 May;61(2):259–66. Review.

36. Birch LL. Psychological influences on the childhood diet. *J Nutr*, 1998 Feb;128 (2 Suppl):407S–10S. Review.

37. Birch LL, et al. Eating as the "means" activity in a contingency: Effects on young children's food preference. *Child Dev*, 1984;55:432–9.

38. Feunekes GI, et al. Food choice and fat intake of adolescents and adults: associations of intakes within social networks. *Prev Med*, 1998 Sep–Oct;27(5 Pt 1): 645–56.

39. Schlundt DG, et al. Obesity: A biogenetic or biobehavioral problem. *Int J Obes*, 1990 Sep;14(9):815–28.

40. Krosnick A. The diabetes and obesity epidemic among the Pima Indians. *N J Med*, 2000 Aug;97(8):31–7.

41. Ravussin E, et al. Effects of a traditional lifestyle on obesity in Pima Indians. *Diabetes Care,* 1994 Sep;17(9):1067–74.

42. Esparza J, et al. Daily energy expenditure in Mexican and USA Pima Indians: Low physical activity as a possible cause of obesity. *Int J Obes Relat Metab Disord,* 2000 Jan;24(1):55–9.

43. Fox C, et al. Plasma leptin concentrations in Pima Indians living in drastically different environments. *Diabetes Care,* 1999 Mar;22(3):413–7.

CHAPTER 4

1. Coppack SW, et al. Adipose tissue metabolism in obesity: Lipase action in vivo before and after a mixed meal. *Metabolism,* 1992 Mar;41(3):264–72.

2. Cusin I, et al. Metabolic consequences of hyperinsulinaemia imposed on normal rats on glucose handling by white adipose tissue, muscles and liver. *Biochem J,* 1990 Apr 1;267(1):99–103.

3. Peterson CM, et al. Randomized crossover study of 40% vs. 55% carbohydrate weight loss strategies in women with previous gestational diabetes mellitus and non-diabetic women of 130–200% ideal body weight. *J Am Coll Nutr,* 1995 Aug;14(4):369–75.

4. Alford BB, et al. The effects of variations in carbohydrate, protein, and fat content of the diet upon weight loss, blood values, and nutrient intake of adult obese women. *J Am Diet Assoc,* 1990 Apr;90(4):534–40.

5. Golay A, et al. Similar weight loss with low- or high-carbohydrate diets. *Am J Clin Nutr,* 1996 Feb;63(2):174–8.

6. Yang MU. Composition of weight lost during short-term weight reduction. Metabolic responses of obese subjects to starvation and low-calorie ketogenic and nonketogenic diets. *J Clin Invest,* 1976 Sep;58(3):722–30.

7. Smith GP, et al. Are gut peptides a new class of anorectic agents? *Am J Clin Nutr,* 1992 Jan;55(1 Suppl):283S–5S. Review.

8. Rolls BJ. Experimental analyses of the effects of variety in a meal on human feeding. *Am J Clin Nutr,* 1985 Nov;42(5 Suppl):932–9.

9. McCrory MA, et al. Dietary variety within food groups: association with energy intake and body fatness in men and women. *Am J Clin Nutr,* 1999 Mar;69(3): 440–7.

10. Filaire E, et al. Food restriction, performance, psychological state and lipid values in judo athletes. *Int J Sports Med,* 2001 Aug;22(6):454–9.

11. Ainslie DA, et al. Short-term, high-fat diets lower circulating leptin concentrations in rats. *Am J Clin Nutr,* 2000 Feb;71(2):438–42.

12. Lin L, et al. Acute changes in the response to peripheral leptin with alteration in the diet composition. *Am J Physiol Regul Integr Comp Physiol,* 2001 Feb;280(2): R504–9.

13. Maughan RJ, et al. The effects of a glycogen-loading regimen on the capacity to perform anaerobic exercise. *Eur J Appl Physiol Occup Physiol,* 1981;46(3):211–9.

14. Jenkins DG, et al. The influence of dietary carbohydrate on performance of supramaximal intermittent exercise. *Eur J Appl Physiol Occup Physiol,* 1993;67(4):309–14.

15. Rooyackers OE, et al. Hormonal regulation of human muscle protein metabolism. *Annu Rev Nutr,* 1997;17:457–85. Review.

16. Wolfe RR. Effects of insulin on muscle tissue. *Curr Opin Clin Nutr Metab Care,* 2000 Jan;3(1):67–71. Review.

17. Marques-Lopes I, et al. Postprandial de novo lipogenesis and metabolic changes induced by a high-carbohydrate, low-fat meal in lean and overweight men. *Am J Clin Nutr,* 2001 Feb;73(2):253–61.

18. Rasmussen O, et al. Comparison of blood glucose and insulin responses in non-insulin-dependent diabetic patients. Studies with spaghetti and potato taken alone and as part of a mixed meal. *Eur J Clin Nutr,* 1988 Nov;42(11):953–61.

19. Gregersen S, et al. Glycaemic and insulinaemic responses to orange and apple compared with white bread in non-insulin-dependent diabetic subjects. *Eur J Clin Nutr,* 1992 Apr;46(4):301–3.

20. Chew I, et al. Application of glycemic index to mixed meals. *Am J Clin Nutr,* 1988 Jan;47(1):53–6.

21. Brand-Miller JC, et al. Glycemic index and obesity. *Am J Clin Nutr,* 2002 Jul;76(1):281S–5S. Review.

22. Slabber M, et al. Effects of a low-insulin-response, energy-restricted diet on weight loss and plasma insulin concentrations in hyperinsulinemic obese females. *Am J Clin Nutr,* 1994;60:48–53.

23. Mannucci E, et al. Clinical features of binge eating disorder in type I diabetes: A case report. *Int J Eat Disord,* 1997 Jan;21(1):99–102.

24. Jenkins DJ, Lente carbohydrate: A newer approach to the dietary management of diabetes. *Diabetes Care,* 1982 Nov–Dec;5(6):634–41.

25. Salmeron J, et al. Dietary fiber, glycemic load, and risk of non-insulin-dependent diabetes mellitus in women. *JAMA,* 1997 Feb 12;277(6):472–7.

26. Slabber M, et al. Effects of a low-insulin-response, energy-restricted diet on weight loss and plasma insulin concentrations in hyperinsulinemic obese females. *Am J Clin Nutr,* 1994 Jul;60(1):48–53.

27. Albrink MJ. Dietary fiber, plasma insulin, and obesity. *Am J Clin Nutr,* 1978 Oct;31(10 Suppl):S277–9.

28. Salmeron J, et al. Dietary fiber, glycemic load, and risk of NIDDM in men. *Diabetes Care,* 1997 Apr;20(4):545–50.

29. Ludwig DS. Dietary glycemic index and obesity. *J Nutr,* 2000 Feb;130(2S Suppl): 280S–3S. Review.

30. Morris KL, et al. Glycemic index, cardiovascular disease, and obesity. *Nutr Rev,* 1999 Sep;57(9 Pt 1):273–6. Review.

31. Hallfrisch J. Metabolic effects of dietary fructose. *FASEB J,* 1990 Jun;4(9):2652–60. Review.

32. Elliott SS, et al. Fructose, weight gain, and the insulin resistance syndrome. *Am J Clin Nutr,* 2002 Nov;76(5):911–22. Review.

33. Howe GR, et al. Dietary intake of fiber and decreased risk of cancers of the colon and rectum: Evidence from the combined analysis of 13 case-control studies. *J Natl Cancer Inst,* 1992 Dec 16;84(24):1887–96.

34. Brown L, et al. Cholesterol-lowering effects of dietary fiber: A meta-analysis. *Am J Clin Nutr,* 1999 Jan;69(1):30–42.

35. Yao M, et al. Dietary energy density and weight regulation. *Nutr Rev,* 2001 Aug;59(8 Pt 1):247–58. Review.

36. Howarth NC, et al. Dietary fiber and weight regulation. *Nutr Rev,* 2001 May;59(5):129–39. Review.

37. Baer, DJ, et al. Dietary fiber decreases the metabolizable energy content and nutrient digestibility of mixed diets fed to humans. *J Nutr,* 1997;127:579–86.

38. Wurtman RJ, et al. Brain serotonin, carbohydrate-craving, obesity and depression. *Obes Res,* 1995 Nov;3 Suppl 4:477S–80S. Review.

39. Rolls BJ. Effects of intense sweeteners on hunger, food intake, and body weight: A review. *Am J Clin Nutr,* 1991 Apr;53(4):872–8.

40. Tordoff MG, et al. Effect of drinking soda sweetened with aspartame or high-fructose corn syrup on food intake and body weight. *Am J Clin Nutr,* 1990 Jun;51(6):963–9.

41. Froff JL, et al. *Advanced Nutrition and Human Metabolism,* 2nd Edition. St Paul: West Publishing Co., 1995.

42. Janssen PJ, et al. Aspartame: Review of recent experimental and observational data. *Toxicology,* 1988 Jun;50(1):1–26.

43. Butchko HH. Acceptable daily intake vs actual intake: The aspartame example. *J Am Coll Nutr,* 1991 Jun;10(3):258–66.

44. Ishii H. Incidence of brain tumors in rats fed aspartame. *Toxicol Lett,* 1981 Mar;7(6):433–7.

45. Renwick AG. The metabolism of intense sweeteners. *Xenobiotica,* 1986 Oct–Nov;16(10–11):1057–71.

46. Walton RG, et al. Adverse reactions to aspartame: Double-blind challenge in patients from a vulnerable population. *Biol Psychiatry,* 1993 Jul 1–15;34(1–2):13–7.

CHAPTER 5

1. Karst H, et al. Diet-induced thermogenesis in man: Thermic effects of single proteins, carbohydrates and fats depending on their energy amount. *Ann Nutr Metab,* 1984;28(4):245–52.

2. De Castro JM. Physiological, environmental, and subjective determinants of food intake in humans: A meal pattern analysis. *Physiol Behav,* 1988;44(4–5):651–9.

3. Porrini M, et al. Evaluation of satiety sensations and food intake after different preloads. *Appetite,* 1995 Aug;25(1):17–30.

4. Moran TH, et al. Gastric and nongastric mechanisms for satiety action of cholecystokinin. *Am J Physiol,* 1988 Apr;254(4 Pt 2):R628–32.

5. Pietrowsky R, et al. Effects of cholecystokinin and calcitonin on evoked brain potentials and satiety in man. *Physiol Behav,* 1989 Sep;46(3):513–19.

6. Paul GL. Dietary protein requirements of physically active individuals. *Sports Med,* 1989 Sep;8(3):154–76.

7. Lemon PW. Protein and amino acid needs of the strength athlete. *Int J Sport Nutr,* 1991 Jun;1(2):127–45. Review.

8. Lemon PW. Do athletes need more dietary protein and amino acids? *Int J Sport Nutr,* 1995 Jun;5 Suppl:S39–61.

9. Henriksson J. Effect of exercise on amino acid concentrations in skeletal muscle and plasma. *J Exp Biol,* 1991 Oct;160:149–65. Review.

10. Walberg JL, et al. Macronutrient content of a hypoenergy diet affects nitrogen retention and muscle function in weight lifters. *Int J Sports Med,* 1988 Aug;9(4): 261–6.

11. Tarnopolsky MA, et al. Evaluation of protein requirements for trained strength athletes. *J Appl Physiol,* 1992 Nov;73(5):1986–95.

12. Blackburn GL. Protein requirements with very low calorie diets. *Postgrad Med J,* 1984;60 Suppl 3:59–65.

13. Castaneda C, et al. Elderly women accommodate to a low-protein diet with losses of body cell mass, muscle function, and immune response. *Am J Clin Nutr,* 1995 Jul;62(1):30–9.

14. Piatti PM, et al. Hypocaloric high-protein diet improves glucose oxidation and spares lean body mass: comparison to hypocaloric high-carbohydrate diet. *Metabolism,* 1994 Dec;43(12):1481–7.

15. Charlton MR, et al. Evidence for a catabolic role of glucagon during an amino acid load. *J Clin Invest,* 1996 Jul 1;98(1):90–9.

16. Takiguchi M, et al. Transcriptional regulation of genes for ornithine cycle enzymes. *Biochem J,* 1995 Dec 15;312 (Pt 3):649–59.

17. Klahr S. Effects of protein intake on the progression of renal disease. *Annu Rev Nutr,* 1989;9:87–108.

18. Millward DJ. Optimal intakes of protein in the human diet. *Proc Nutr Soc,* 1999 May;58(2):403–13.

19. Manz F, et al. Effects of a high protein intake on renal acid excretion in bodybuilders. *Z Ernahrungswiss,* 1995 Mar;34(1):10–15.

20. Skov AR, et al. Changes in renal function during weight loss induced by high vs low-protein low-fat diets in overweight subjects. *Int J Obes Relat Metab Disord,* 1999 Nov;23(11):1170–7.

21. Knight EL, et al. The impact of protein intake on renal function decline in women with normal renal function or mild renal insufficiency. *Ann Intern Med,* 2003 Mar 18;138(6):460–7.

22. Poortmans JR, et al. Do regular high protein diets have potential health risks on kidney function in athletes? *Int J Sport Nutr Exerc Metab,* 2000 Mar;10(1):28–38.

23. Metz JA, et al. A randomized trial of improved weight loss with a prepared meal plan in overweight and obese patients: Impact on cardiovascular risk reduction. *Arch Intern Med,* 2000 Jul;160(14):2150–8.

24. Bujko J, et al. Benefit of more but smaller meals at a fixed daily protein intake. *Z Ernahrungswiss,* 1997 Dec;36(4):347–9.

25. Desenclos JC. Epidemiology of toxic and infectious risk related to shellfish consumption. *Rev Epidemiol Sante Publique,* 1996 Oct;44(5):437–54. Review. French.

26. Killduff LP, et al. Effects of creatine on isometric bench-press performance in resistance-trained humans. *Med Sci Sports Exerc,* 2002 Jul;34(7):1176–83.

27. Demant TW, et al. Effects of creatine supplementation on exercise performance. *Sports Med,* 1999 Jul;28(1):49–60. Review.

28. Clarkson TB. Soy, soy phytoestrogens and cardiovascular disease. *J Nutr,* 2002 Mar;132(3):566S–9S. Review.

29. Nagata C, et al. Hot flushes and other menopausal symptoms in relation to soy product intake in Japanese women. *Climacteric,* 1999 Mar;2(1):6–12.

30. Chiechi LM, et al. Efficacy of a soy rich diet in preventing postmenopausal osteoporosis: The Menfis randomized trial. *Maturitas,* 2002 Aug 30;42(4):295–300.

31. Han KK, et al. Benefits of soy isoflavone therapeutic regimen on menopausal symptoms. *Obstet Gynecol,* 2002 Mar;99(3):389–94.

32. Scheiber MD, et al. Dietary inclusion of whole soy foods results in significant reductions in clinical risk factors for osteoporosis and cardiovascular disease in normal postmenopausal women. *Menopause,* 2001 Sep–Oct;8(5):384–92.

33. Arliss RM, et al. Do soy isoflavones lower cholesterol, inhibit atherosclerosis, and play a role in cancer prevention? *Holist Nurs Pract,* 2002 Oct;16(5):40–8. Review.

34. Allred CD, et al. Dietary genistin stimulates growth of estrogen-dependent breast cancer tumors similar to that observed with genistein. *Carcinogenesis,* 2001 Oct;22(10):1667–73.

35. Yellayi S, et al. The phytoestrogen genistein induces thymic and immune changes: A human health concern? *Proc Natl Acad Sci USA,* 2002 May 28;99(11): 7616–21.

36. Molis CB, et al. Digestion, excretion, and energy value of fructooligosaccharides in healthy humans. *Am J Clin Nutr,* 1996 Sep;64(3):324–8.

CHAPTER 6

1. Harvey-Berino J. The efficacy of dietary fat vs. total energy restriction for weight loss. *Obes Res,* 1998 May;6(3):202–7.

2. Horton TJ, et al. Fat and carbohydrate overfeeding in humans: Different effects on energy storage. *Am J Clin Nutr,* 1995 Jul;62(1):19–29.

3. Romieu I, et al. Energy intake and other determinants of relative weight. *Am J Clin Nutr,* 1988 Mar;47(3):406–12.

4. Tholstrup T, et al. Fat high in stearic acid favorably affects blood lipids and factor VII coagulant activity in comparison with fats high in palmitic acid or high in myristic and lauric acids. *Am J Clin Nutr* 1994;59:371–7.

5. Engstrom G, et al. Long-term effects of inflammation-sensitive plasma proteins and systolic blood pressure on incidence of stroke. *Stroke,* 2002 Dec;33(12): 2744–9.

6. Stucchi AF, et al. LDL receptor activity is down-regulated similarly by a cholesterol-containing diet high in palmitic acid or high in lauric and myristic acids in cynomolgus monkeys. *J Nutr,* 1995 Aug;125(8):2055–63.

7. Nicolosi RJ. Dietary fat saturation effects on low-density-lipoprotein concentrations and metabolism in various animal models. *Am J Clin Nutr,* 1997 May;65 (5 Suppl):1617S–27S. Review.

8. Kesteloot H, et al. Cancer mortality and age: Relationship with dietary fat. *Nutr Cancer,* 1994;22(1):85–98.

9. La Vecchia C, et al. Monounsaturated and other types of fat, and the risk of breast cancer. *Eur J Cancer Prev,* 1998 Dec;7(6):461–4.

10. Bairati I, et al. Dietary fat and advanced prostate cancer. *J Urol,* 1998 Apr;159(4): 1271–5.

11. Riboli E, et al. Diet and bladder cancer in Spain: A multi-centre case-control study. *Int J Cancer,* 1991 Sep 9;49(2):214–9.

12. Yang G, et al. Dietary factors and cancer of the colon and rectum in a population based case-control study in Shanghai. *Zhonghua Liu Xing Bing Xue Za Zhi,* 1994 Oct;15(5):299–303.

13. Miller AB, et al. Food items and food groups as risk factors in a case-control study of diet and colon cancer. *Int. J. Cancer,* 1983;32:155–62.

14. Giovannucci E, et al. Dietary factors and risk of colon cancer. *Ann Med,* 1994;26:443–52.

15. Marshall JA, et al. High saturated fat and low starch and fibre are associated with hyperinsulinaemia in a non-diabetic population: The San Luis Valley Diabetes Study. *Diabetologia,* 1997 Apr;40(4):430–8.

16. Rivellese AA, et al. Type of dietary fat and insulin resistance. *Ann NY Acad Sci,* 2002 Jun;967:329–35. Review.

17. Havel PJ, et al. High-fat meals reduce 24-h circulating leptin concentrations in women. *Diabetes,* 1999 Feb;48(2):334–41.

18. Stark AH, et al. Olive oil as a functional food: Epidemiology and nutritional approaches. *Nutr Rev,* 2002 Jun;60(6):170–6. Review.

19. Owen RW, et al. Olive-oil consumption and health: The possible role of antioxidants. *Lancet Oncol,* 2000 Oct;1:107–12. Review.

20. Trichopoulou A. Mediterranean diet: The past and the present. *Nutr Metab Cardiovasc Dis,* 2001 Aug;11(4 Suppl):1–4.

21. Sanders TA. Olive oil and the Mediterranean diet. *Int J Vitam Nutr Res,* 2001 May;71(3):179–84. Review.

22. Piers LS, et al. The influence of the type of dietary fat on postprandial fat oxidation rates: monounsaturated (olive oil) vs saturated fat (cream). *Int J Obes Relat Metab Disord,* 2002 Jun;26(6):814–21.

23. von Schacky C. N-3 fatty acids and the prevention of coronary atherosclerosis. *Am J Clin Nutr,* 2000 Jan;71(1 Suppl):224S–7S.

24. Connor WE, et al. N-3 fatty acids from fish oil. Effects on plasma lipoproteins and hypertriglyceridemic patients. *Ann NY Acad Sci,* 1993 Jun 14;683: 16–34.

25. Lindgren FT, et al. Effect of a salmon diet on the distribution of plasma lipoproteins and apolipoproteins in normolipidemic adult men. *Lipids,* 1991 Feb;26(2): 97–101.

26. de Lorgeril M, et al. Mediterranean alpha-linolenic acid-rich diet in secondary prevention of coronary heart disease. *Lancet,* 1994 Jun 11;343(8911):1454–9.

27. DeLany J, et al. Differential oxidation of individual dietary fatty acids in humans. *Am J Clin Nutr,* 2000;72:905–11.

28. Raclot T, et al. Site-specific regulation of gene expression by n-3 polyunsaturated fatty acids in rat white adipose tissues. *J Lipid Res,* 1997 Oct;38(10):1963–72.

29. Sadurskis A, et al. Polyunsaturated fatty acids recruit brown adipose tissue: Increased UCP content and NST capacity. *Am J Physiol,* 1995 Aug;269(2 Pt 1): E351–60.

30. Schrauwen P, et al. Human uncoupling proteins and obesity. *Obes Res,* 1999 Jan;7(1):97–105. Review.

31. Cha MC, et al. Dietary fat type and energy restriction interactively influence plasma leptin concentration in rats. *J Lipid Res,* 1998 Aug;39(8):1655–60.

32. Eaton SB, et al. Paleolithic nutrition. A consideration of its nature and current implications. *N Engl J Med,* 1985 Jan 31;312(5):283–9. Review.

33. Simopoulos AP. Evolutionary aspects of omega-3 fatty acids in the food supply. *Prostaglandins Leukot Essent Fatty Acids,* 1999 May–Jun;60(5–6):421–9. Review.

34. Davidson M, et al. Cardiac mortality in Alaska's indigenous and non-Native residents. *Int J Epidemiol,* 1993 Feb;22(1):62–71.

35. Feskens EJ, et al. Epidemiologic studies on Eskimos and fish intake. *NY Acad Sci,* 1993 Jun 14;683:9–15. Review.

36. Gillman MW, et al. Margarine intake and subsequent coronary heart disease in men. *Epidemiology,* 1997 Mar;8(2):144–9.

37. Mann GV. Metabolic consequences of dietary trans fatty acids. *Lancet,* 1994 May 21;343(8908):1268–71.

38. Ascherio A, et al. Health effects of trans fatty acids. *Am J Clin Nutr,* 1997;66: 1006S–10S.

39. Booyens J, et al. Margarines and coronary artery disease. *Med Hypotheses,* 1992 Apr;37(4):241–4. Review.

40. Slattery ML, et al. Trans-fatty acids and colon cancer. *Nutr Cancer,* 2001; 39(2):170–5.

41. Trans fatty acids and coronary heart disease risk. Report of the expert panel on trans fatty acids and coronary heart disease. *Am J Clin Nutr,* 1995 Sep;62(3): 655S–708S.

CHAPTER 7

1. Anastasio P, et al. Level of hydration and renal function in healthy humans. *Kidney Int,* 2001 Aug;60(2):748–56.

2. Bankir L, et al. Is the process of urinary urea concentration responsible for a high glomerular filtration rate? *J Am Soc Nephrol,* 1993 Nov;4(5):1091–103.

3. Lappalainen R, et al. Drinking water with a meal: A simple method of coping with feelings of hunger, satiety and desire to eat. *Eur J Clin Nutr,* 1993;47:815–9.

4. Michaud DS, et al. Fluid intake and the risk of bladder cancer in men. *N Engl J Med,* 1999 May 6;340(18):1390–7.

5. Shannon J, et al. Relationship of food groups and water intake to colon cancer risk. *Cancer Epidemiol Biomarkers Prev,* 1996 Jul;5(7):495–502.

6. Tang R, et al. Physical activity, water intake and risk of colorectal cancer in Taiwan: A hospital-based case-control study. *Int J Cancer,* 1999 Aug 12;82(4):484–9.

7. Lubin F, et al. Nutritional and lifestyle habits and water-fiber interaction in colorectal adenoma etiology. *Cancer Epidemiol Biomarkers Prev,* 1997 Feb;6(2): 79–85.

8. Chan J, et al. Water, other fluids, and fatal coronary heart disease: The Adventist Health Study. *Am J Epidemiol,* 2002 May 1;155(9):827–33.

9. Brunner FP. Pathophysiology of dehydration. *Schweiz Rundsch Med Prax,* 1993 Jul 20;82(29–30):784–7.

10. Choukroun G, et al. Low urine flow reduces the capacity to excrete a sodium load in humans. *Am J Physiol,* 1997 Nov;273(5 Pt 2):R1726–33.

11. Churchill TA, et al. Metabolic effects of dehydration on an aquatic frog, *Rana pipiens. J Exp Biol,* 1995 Jan;198 (Pt 1):147–54.

12. Loria CM, et al. Choose and prepare foods with less salt: dietary advice for all Americans. *J Nutr,* 2001 Feb;131(2S-1):536S–51S.

13. Sulyok E, et al. Renal aspects of neonatal sodium homeostasis. *Acta Paediatr Hung* 1983;24(1):23–35.

14. Valtin H, et al. *Renal Function Mechanisms Preserving Fluid and Solute Balance in Health,* 3rd Edition. Boston: Little, Brown, 1995.

15. Kleiner SM. Water: An essential but overlooked nutrient. *J Am Diet Assoc,* 1999 Feb;99(2):200–6. Review.

16. Grandjean AC, et al. The effect of caffeinated, non-caffeinated, caloric and non-caloric beverages on hydration. *J Am Coll Nutr,* 2000 Oct;19(5):591–600.

17. Shirreffs SM, et al. Restoration of fluid balance after exercise-induced dehydration: Effects of alcohol consumption. *J Appl Physiol,* 1997 Oct;83(4):1152–8.

18. Roberts, KE. Mechanism of dehydration following alcohol ingestion. *Arch Intern Med,* 1963;112:154–7.

19. Klonoff DC, et al. Acute water intoxication as a complication of urine drug testing in the workplace. *JAMA,* 1991 Jan 2;265(1):84–5. Review.

20. Bove F, et al. Drinking water contaminants and adverse pregnancy outcomes: A review. *Environ Health Perspect,* 2002 Feb;110 Suppl 1:61–74. Review.

21. Cantor KP. Drinking water and cancer. *Cancer Causes Control,* 1997 May;8(3):292–308.

22. Magnus P, et al. Water chlorination and birth defects. *Epidemiology,* 1999 Sep;10(5):513–7.

23. Calderon RL, The epidemiology of chemical contaminants of drinking water. *Food Chem Toxicol,* 2000;38(1 Suppl):S13–20.

24. Page BD, et al. Survey of bottled drinking water sold in Canada. Part 2. Selected volatile organic compounds. *J AOAC Int,* 1993 Jan–Feb;76(1):26–31.

25. Dabeka RW, et al. Survey of bottled drinking waters sold in Canada for chlorate, bromide, bromate, lead, cadmium and other trace elements. *Food Addit Contam,* 2002 Aug;19(8):721–32.

26. Misund A, et al. Variation of 66 elements in European bottled mineral waters. *Sci Total Environ,* 1999 Dec 15;243–44:21–41.

CHAPTER 8

1. Oscai LB. The role of exercise in weight control. *Exerc Sport Sci Rev,* 1973; 1:103–23.

2. Elliot DL, et al. Sustained depression of the resting metabolic rate after massive weight loss. *Am J Clin Nutr,* 1989 Jan;49(1):93–6.

3. Kern PA, et al. The effects of weight loss on the activity and expression of adipose-tissue lipoprotein lipase in very obese humans. *N Engl J Med,* 1990 Apr 12;322(15):1053–9.

4. Moore R, et al. The role of T3 and its receptor in efficient metabolisers receiving very-low-calorie diets. *Int J Obes,* 1981;5(3):283–6.

5. Welle SL, et al. Decrease in resting metabolic rate during rapid weight loss is reversed by low dose thyroid hormone treatment. *Metabolism,* 1986 Apr;35(4): 289–91.

6. Brownell KD, et al. The effect of repeated cycles of weight loss and regain in rats. *Physiol Behav,* 1986;38:459–64.

7. Brownell KD, et al. Medical, metabolic and psychological effects of weight cycling. *Arch Intern Med,* 1994;154:1325–30.

8. Muls E, et al. Is weight cycling detrimental to health? A review of literature in humans. *Int J Obes Relat Metab Disord,* 1995;19:S46–50.

9. Jen KL, et al. Long-term weight cycling reduces body weight and fat free mass, but not fat mass in female Wistar rats. *Int J Obes Relat Metab Disord,* 1995 Oct;19(10):699–708.

10. Kolaczynski JW, et al. Response of leptin to short-term and prolonged overfeeding in humans. *J Clin Endocrinol Metab,* 1996 Nov;81(11):4162–5.

11. Saladin R, et al. Transient increase in obese gene expression after food intake or insulin administration. *Nature,* 1995 Oct 12;377(6549):527–9.

12. Kolaczynski JW, et al. Responses of leptin to short-term fasting and refeeding in humans: A link with ketogenesis but not ketones themselves. *Diabetes,* 1996 Nov;45(11):1511–5.

13. Havel PJ, et al. Relationship of plasma leptin to plasma insulin and adiposity in normal weight and overweight women: Effects of dietary fat content and sustained weight loss. *J Clin Endocrinol Metab,* 1996 Dec;81(12):4406–13.

14. Bado A, et al. The stomach is a source of leptin. *Nature,* 1998 Aug 20;394(6695): 790–3.

15. Friedman JM, et al. Leptin and the regulation of body weight in mammals. *Nature,* 1998 Oct 22;395(6704):763–70. Review.

16. Wisse BE, et al. Effect of prolonged moderate and severe energy restriction and refeeding on plasma leptin concentrations in obese women. *Am J Clin Nutr,* 1999 Sep;70(3):321–30.

17. Kolaczynski JW, et al. Response of leptin to short-term and prolonged overfeeding in humans. *J Clin Endocrinol Metab*, 1996 Nov;81(11):4162–5.

18. Dirlewanger M, et al. Effects of short-term carbohydrate or fat overfeeding on energy expenditure and plasma leptin concentrations in healthy female subjects. *Int J Obes Relat Metab Disord*, 2000 Nov;24(11):1413–8.

19. Levin BE, et al. Defense of differing body weight set points in diet-induced obese and resistant rats. *Am J Physiol*, 1998 Feb;274(2 Pt 2):R412–9.

20. Flatt JP. The biochemistry of energy expenditure. In: *Recent Advances in Obesity Research II*, edited by G. Bray. London: Libbey, 1980, pp. 211–18.

21. Jequier E, et al. Energy expenditure in obesity and diabetes. *Diabetes Metab Rev*, 1988 Sep;4(6):583–93. Review.

CHAPTER 9

1. Rogers PJ. Eating habits and appetite control: A psychobiological perspective. *Proc Nutr Soc*, 1999 Feb;58(1):59–67. Review.

2. Kmiec Z, et al. Thyroid hormones homeostasis in rats refed after short-term and prolonged fasting. *J Endocrinol Invest*, 1996 May;19(5):304–11.

3. Jenkins DJ, et al. Metabolic advantages of spreading the nutrient load: Effects of increased meal frequency in non-insulin-dependent diabetes. *Am J Clin Nutr*, 1992 Feb;55(2):461–7.

4. Speechly DP, et al. Acute appetite reduction associated with an increased frequency of eating in obese males. *Int J Obes Relat Metab Disord*, 1999 Nov; 23(11):1151–9.

5. Speechly DP, et al. Greater appetite control associated with an increased frequency of eating in lean males. *Appetite*, 1999 Dec;33(3):285–97.

6. Deutz RC, et al. Relationship between energy deficits and body composition in elite female gymnasts and runners. *Med Sci Sports Exerc*, 2000 Mar;32(3):659–68.

7. LeBlanc J, et al. Effect of meal size and frequency on postprandial thermogenesis in dogs. *Am J Physiol*, 1986 Feb;250(2 Pt 1):E144–7.

8. LeBlanc J, et al. Components of postprandial thermogenesis in relation to meal frequency in humans. *Can J Physiol Pharmacol*, 1993 Dec;71(12):879–83.

9. Iwao S, et al. Effects of meal frequency on body composition during weight control in boxers. *Scand J Med Sci Sports*, 1996 Oct;6(5):265–72.

10. Antoine JM. Feeding frequency and nitrogen balance in weight-reducing obese women. *Hum Nutr Clin Nutr,* 1984 Jan;38(1):31–8.

11. Ortega RM, et al. Relationship between the number of daily meals and the energy and nutrient intake in the elderly. Effect on various cardiovascular risk factors. *Nutr Hosp,* 1998 Jul–Aug;13(4):186–92.

12. McGrath SA, et al. The effects of altered frequency of eating on plasma lipids in free-living healthy males on normal self-selected diets. *Eur J Clin Nutr,* 1994 Jun;48(6):402–7.

13. Arnold LM, et al. Effect of isoenergetic intake of three or nine meals on plasma lipoproteins and glucose metabolism. *Am J Clin Nutr,* 1993 Mar;57(3):446–51.

14. Powell JT, et al. Does nibbling or grazing protect the peripheral arteries from atherosclerosis? *J Cardiovasc Risk,* 1999 Feb;6(1):19–22.

15. Ashley JM, et al. Meal replacements in weight intervention. *Obes Res,* 2001 Nov;9 Suppl 4:312S–20S.

16. Quinn Rothacker D. Five-year self-management of weight using meal replacements: Comparison with matched controls in rural Wisconsin. *Nutrition,* 2000 May;16(5):344–8.

17. Acheson KJ. Glycogen storage capacity and de novo lipogenesis during massive carbohydrate overfeeding in man. *Am J Clin Nutr,* 1988 Aug;48(2):240–7.

18. Lee A, et al. Diurnal variation in glucose tolerance. Cyclic suppression of insulin action and insulin secretion in normal-weight, but not obese, subjects. *Diabetes,* 1992 Jun;41(6):742–9.

19. Morgan LM, et al. Diurnal variations in peripheral insulin resistance and plasma non-esterified fatty acid concentrations: A possible link? *Ann Clin Biochem,* 1999 Jul;36 (Pt 4):447–50.

20. Wolever TM, et al. Second-meal effect: Low-glycemic-index foods eaten at dinner improve subsequent breakfast glycemic response. *Am J Clin Nutr,* 1988 Oct;48(4):1041–7.

21. Latner JD, et al. The effects of a high-carbohydrate, high-protein or balanced lunch upon later food intake and hunger ratings. *Appetite,* 1999 Aug;33(1): 119–28.

22. Weisburger JH. Comments on the history and importance of aromatic and heterocyclic amines in public health. *Mutat Res,* 2002 Sep 30;506–7:9–20.

23. Salmon CP, et al. Effects of marinating on heterocyclic amine carcinogen formation in grilled chicken. *Food Chem Toxicol*, 1997 May;35(5):433–41.

24. Felton JS, et al. Effect of microwave pretreatment on heterocyclic aromatic amine mutagens/carcinogens in fried beef patties. *Food Chem Toxicol*, 1994 Oct;32(10):897–903.

25. Salmon CP, et al. Minimization of heterocyclic amines and thermal inactivation of *Escherichia coli* in fried ground beef. *J Natl Cancer Inst*, 2000 Nov 1;92(21):1773–8.

26. Gere A. Decrease in essential fatty acid content of edible fats during the frying process. *Z Ernahrungswiss*, 1982 Sep;21(3):191–201.

27. Durak I, et al. High-temperature effects on antioxidant systems and toxic product formation in nutritional oils. *J Toxicol Environ Health*, 1999 Aug 27;57(8): 585–9.

28. Knize MG, et al. Mutagenic activity and heterocyclic amine content of the human diet. *Princess Takamatsu Symp*, 1995;23:30–8. Review.

29. Zock PL, et al. Dietary trans-fatty acids: A risk factor for coronary disease. *Ned Tijdschr Geneeskd*, 1998 Jul 25;142(30):1701–4. Review.

30. Fillion L, et al. Nutrient losses and gains during frying: A review. *Int J Food Sci Nutr*, 1998 Mar;49(2):157–68. Review.

31. Heath JL, et al. Migration of acetyl-tributylcitrate from plastic film into poultry products during microwave cooking. *Poult Sci*, 1981 Oct;60(10):2258–64.

32. Stubbs J, et al. Energy density of foods: effects on energy intake. *Crit Rev Food Sci Nutr*, 2000 Nov;40(6):481–515. Review.

33. Orozco S, et al. Effects of alcohol abstinence on spontaneous feeding patterns in moderate alcohol consuming humans. *Pharmacol Biochem Behav*, 1991 Dec;40(4):867–73.

34. De Castro JM, et al. Moderate alcohol intake and spontaneous eating patterns of humans: Evidence of unregulated supplementation. *Am J Clin Nutr*, 1990 Aug;52(2):246–53.

35. Suter PM, et al. The effect of ethanol on fat storage in healthy subjects. *N Engl J Med*, 1992 Apr 9;326(15):983–7.

36. Murgatroyd PR, et al. Alcohol and the regulation of energy balance: Overnight effects on diet-induced thermogenesis and fuel storage. *Br J Nutr*, 1996 Jan;75(1):33–45.

37. Heikkonen E, et al. The combined effect of alcohol and physical exercise on serum testosterone, luteinizing hormone, and cortisol in males. *Alcohol Clin Exp Res*, 1996 Jun;20(4):711–6.

38. Reilly ME, et al. Studies on the time-course of ethanol's acute effects on skeletal muscle protein synthesis: Comparison with acute changes in proteolytic activity. *Alcohol Clin Exp Res*, 1997 Aug;21(5):792–8.

38. Preedy VR, et al. The acute effects of ethanol and acetaldehyde on rates of protein synthesis in type I and type II fibre-rich skeletal muscles of the rat. *Alcohol*, 1992 May;27(3):241–51.

40. Hodges DL, et al. Effects of alcohol on bone, muscle and nerve. *Am Fam Physician*, 1986 Nov;34(5):149–56.

41. Das DK, et al. Cardioprotection of red wine: Role of polyphenolic antioxidants. *Drugs Exp Clin Res*, 1999;25(2–3):115–20. Review.

42. Sato M, et al. Cardioprotection with alcohol: Role of both alcohol and polyphenolic antioxidants. *Ann NY Acad Sci*, 2002 May;957:122–35.

43. Pike MC, et al. Statistical errors invalidate conclusions in "Caffeine and unsaturated fat diet significantly promotes DMBA-induced breast cancer in rats." *Cancer*, 1985 Apr 15;55(8):1855–8.

44. Pozniak PC. The carcinogenicity of caffeine and coffee: A review. *J Am Diet Assoc*, 1985 Sep;85(9):1127–33.

45. Phelps HM, et al. Caffeine ingestion and breast cancer. A negative correlation. *Cancer*, 1988 Mar 1;61(5):1051–4.

46. Leonard TK, et al. The effects of caffeine on various body systems: A review. *J Am Diet Assoc*, 1987 Aug;87(8):1048–53. Review.

47. Jung RT, et al. Caffeine: Its effect on catecholamines and metabolism in lean and obese humans. *Clin Sci*, 1981 May;60(5):527–35.

48. Acheson KJ, et al. Caffeine and coffee: Their influence on metabolic rate and substrate utilization in normal weight and obese individuals. *Am J Clin Nutr*, 1980 May;33(5):989–97.

49. Astrup A, et al. Caffeine: A double-blind, placebo-controlled study of its thermogenic, metabolic, and cardiovascular effects in healthy volunteers. *Am J Clin Nutr*, 1990 May;51(5):759–67.

50. Baldessarini RJ, et al. Inhibition of catechol-O-methyl transferase by catechols and polyphenols. *Biochem Pharmacol*, 1973 Jan 15;22(2):247–56.

51. Dulloo AG, et al. Green tea and thermogenesis: Interactions between catechin-polyphenols, caffeine and sympathetic activity. *Int J Obes Relat Metab Disord,* 2000 Feb;24(2):252–8.

52. Wu CH, et al. Epidemiological evidence of increased bone mineral density in habitual tea drinkers. *Arch Intern Med,* 2002 May 13;162(9):1001–6.

53. Geleijnse JM, et al. Inverse association of tea and flavonoid intakes with incident myocardial infarction: The Rotterdam Study. *Am J Clin Nutr,* 2002 May;75(5):880–6.

54. Valdez IH, et al. Interactions of the salivary and gastrointestinal systems. I. The role of saliva in digestion. *Dig Dis,* 1991;9(3):125–32. Review.

55. Duncan KH, et al. The effects of high and low energy density diets on satiety, energy intake, and eating time of obese and nonobese subjects. *Am J Clin Nutr,* 1983;37:763–7.

56. Jordan HA, et al. Role of food characteristics in behavioral change and weight loss. *J Am Diet Assoc,* 1981;79:24–9.

57. Spiegel TA, et al. Objective measurement of eating rate during behavioral treatment of obesity. *Behav Ther,* 1991;22:61–7.

58. Laporte DJ. Influences of gender, amount of food, and speed of eating on external raters' perceptions of binge eating. *Appetite,* 1996 Apr;26(2):119–27.

59. Liljeberg H, et al. Delayed gastric emptying rate may explain improved glycaemia in healthy subjects to a starchy meal with added vinegar. *Eur J Clin Nutr,* 1998 May;52(5):368–71.

60. Osaka T, et al. Thermogenesis mediated by a capsaicin-sensitive area in the ventrolateral medulla. *Neuroreport,* 2000 Aug 3;11(11):2425–8.

61. Ohnuki K, et al. Administration of capsiate, a non-pungent capsaicin analog, promotes energy metabolism and suppresses body fat accumulation in mice. *Biosci Biotechnol Biochem,* 2001 Dec;65(12):2735–40.

62. Yoshioka M, et al. Effects of red pepper on appetite and energy intake. *Br J Nutr,* 1999 Aug;82(2):115–23.

63. Eldershaw TP, et al. Pungent principles of ginger (*Zingiber officinale*) are thermogenic in the perfused rat hindlimb. *Int J Obes Relat Metab Disord,* 1992 Oct;16(10):755–63.

64. Mazzeo-Caputo SE, et al. Dietary change: Prescription vs. goal setting. *J Am Diet Assoc,* 1985 May;85(5):553–6.

65. Coates TJ, et al. Heart healthy eating and exercise: Introducing and maintaining changes in health behaviors. *Am J Public Health*, 1981 Jan;71(1):15–23.

66. De Castro JM. Independence of heritable influences on the food intake of free-living humans. *Nutrition*, 2002 Jan;18(1):11–6; discussion 91–2.

CHAPTER 10

1. Treuth MS, et al. Effects of exercise intensity on 24-h energy expenditure and substrate oxidation. *Med Sci Sports Exerc*, 1996 Sep;28(9):1138–43.

2. Schuenke MD, et al. Effect of an acute period of resistance exercise on excess post-exercise oxygen consumption: implications for body mass management. *Eur J Appl Physiol*, 2002 Mar;86(5):411–7.

3. Despres JP. Visceral obesity, insulin resistance, and dyslipidemia: Contribution of endurance exercise training to the treatment of the plurimetabolic syndrome. *Exerc Sport Sci Rev*, 1997;25:271–300. Review.

4. Chu NF, et al. Dietary and lifestyle factors in relation to plasma leptin concentrations among normal weight and overweight men. *Int J Obes Relat Metab Disord*, 2001 Jan;25(1):106–14.

5. Long SJ, et al. The ability of habitual exercise to influence appetite and food intake in response to high- and low-energy preloads in man. *Br J Nutr*, 2002 May; 87(5):517–23.

6. Cavagnini F, et al. Glucocorticoids and neuroendocrine function. *Int J Obes Relat Metab Disord*, 2000 Jun;24 Suppl 2:S77–9. Review.

7. Ottosson M, et al. The effects of cortisol on the regulation of lipoprotein lipase activity in human adipose tissue. *J Clin Endocrinol Metab*, 1994 Sep;79(3):820–5.

8. Solano JM, et al. Glucocorticoids reverse leptin effects on food intake and body fat in mice without increasing NPY mRNA. *Am J Physiol*, 1999 Oct;277(4 Pt 1):E708–16.

9. Zakrzewska KE, et al. Glucocorticoids as counterregulatory hormones of leptin: Toward an understanding of leptin resistance. *Diabetes*, 1997 Apr;46(4):717–9.

10. Björntorp P. Do stress reactions cause abdominal obesity and comorbidities? *Obes Rev*, 2001 May;2(2):73–86.

11. Wigers SH, et al. Effects of aerobic exercise versus stress management treatment in fibromyalgia. A 4.5 year prospective study. *Scand J Rheumatol*, 1996;25(2): 77–86.

12. Schwarz L, et al. Changes in beta-endorphin levels in response to aerobic and anaerobic exercise. *Sports Med,* 1992 Jan;13(1):25–36. Review.

13. Thorell A, et al. Exercise and insulin cause GLUT-4 translocation in human skeletal muscle. *Am J Physiol,* 1999 Oct;277(4 Pt 1):E733–41.

14. Zurlo F, et al. Skeletal muscle metabolism is a major determinant of resting energy expenditure. *J Clin Invest,* 1990 Nov;86(5):1423–7.

15. Hammer RL, et al. Calorie-restricted low-fat diet and exercise in obese women. *Am J Clin Nutr,* 1989 Jan;49(1):77–85.

16. Bryner RW, et al. Effects of resistance vs. aerobic training combined with an 800 calorie liquid diet on lean body mass and resting metabolic rate. *J Am Coll Nutr,* 1999 Apr;18(2):115–21.

17. Donnelly JE, et al. Muscle hypertrophy with large-scale weight loss and resistance training. *Am J Clin Nutr,* 1993 Oct;58(4):561–5.

18. Ballor DL, et al. Resistance weight training during caloric restriction enhances lean body weight maintenance. *Am J Clin Nutr,* 1988 Jan;47(1):19–25.

19. Tipton KD, et al. Timing of amino acid-carbohydrate ingestion alters anabolic response of muscle to resistance exercise. *Am J Physiol Endocrinol Metab,* 2001 Aug;281(2):E197–206.

20. Maffucci DM, et al. Towards optimizing the timing of the pre-exercise meal. *Int J Sport Nutr Exerc Metab,* 2000 Jun;10(2):103–13.

21. Walton P, et al. Glycaemic index and optimal performance. *Sports Med,* 1997 Mar;23(3):164–72. Review.

22. Kuipers H, et al. Pre-exercise ingestion of carbohydrate and transient hypoglycemia during exercise. *Int J Sports Med,* 1999 May;20(4):227–31.

23. Decombaz J, et al. Oxidation and metabolic effects of fructose or glucose ingested before exercise. *Int J Sports Med,* 1985 Oct;6(5):282–6.

24. Dangin M, et al. The digestion rate of protein is an independent regulating factor of postprandial protein retention. *Am J Physiol Endocrinol Metab,* 2001 Feb; 280(2):340E–8E.

25. Jung RT, et al. Caffeine: Its effect on catecholamines and metabolism in lean and obese humans. *Clin Sci,* 1981 May;60(5):527–35.

26. Graham TE. Caffeine and exercise: Metabolism, endurance and performance. *Sports Med,* 2001;31(11):785–807. Review.

27. Barr SI. Effects of dehydration on exercise performance. *Can J Appl Physiol*, 1999 Apr;24(2):164–72.

28. Costill DL, et al. Nutrition for endurance sport. Carbohydrate and fluid balance. *Int J Sports Med*, 1980;1:2–14.

29. Mack GW, et al. Body fluid balance in dehydrated healthy older men: Thirst and renal osmoregulation. *J Appl Physiol*, 1994 Apr;76(4):1615–23.

30. Latzka WA, et al. Water and electrolyte requirements for exercise. *Clin Sports Med*, 1999 Jul;18(3):513–24.

31. Anantaraman R, et al. Effects of carbohydrate supplementation on performance during 1 hour of high-intensity exercise. *Int J Sports Med.* 1995 Oct;16(7):461.

32. Convertino VA, et al. American College of Sports Medicine position stand. Exercise and fluid replacement. *Med Sci Sports Exerc*, 1996 Jan;28(1):i–vii. Review.

33. Donal J, et al. Insulin and exercise differentially regulate PI3-kinase and glycogen synthase in human skeletal muscle. *J Appl Physiol*, 2000;89:1412–19.

34. Fluckey JD, et al. Augmented insulin action on rates of protein synthesis after resistance exercise in rats. *Am J Physiol*, 1996 Feb;270(2 Pt 1):E313–19.

35. Katz J, et al. The glucose paradox. Is glucose a substrate for liver metabolism? *J Clin Invest*, 1984 Dec;74(6):1901–9. Review.

36. Ivy JL. Glycogen resynthesis after exercise: Effect of carbohydrate intake. *Int J Sports Med*, 1998 Jun;19 Suppl 2:S142–5.

37. Rasmussen BB, et al. An oral essential amino acid-carbohydrate supplement enhances muscle protein anabolism after resistance exercise. *J Appl Physiol*, 2000 Feb;88(2):386–92.

38. Thong FS, et al. Caffeine-induced impairment of insulin action but not insulin signaling in human skeletal muscle is reduced by exercise. *Diabetes*, 2002 Mar;51(3):583–90.

39. Esmarck B, et al. Timing of postexercise protein intake is important for muscle hypertrophy with resistance training in elderly humans. *Journal of Physiology*, 2001;535.1:301–11.

CHAPTER 11

1. McCrory MA, et al. Dietary determinants of energy intake and weight regulation in healthy adults. *J Nutr*, 2000 Feb;130(2S Suppl):276S–9S. Review.

2. Guthri JF, et al. Role of food prepared away from home in the American diet, 1977–78 versus 1994–96: Changes and consequences. *J Nutr Educ Behav,* 2002 May–Jun;34(3):140–50.

CHAPTER 12

1. Chan ST, et al. Early weight gain and glycogen-obligated water during nutritional rehabilitation. *Hum Nutr Clin Nutr,* 1982;36(3):223–32.

2. Geliebter A, et al. Overfeeding with medium-chain triglyceride diet results in diminished deposition of fat. *Am J Clin Nutr,* 1983 Jan;37(1):1–4.

3. Jeukendrup AE, et al. Fat metabolism during exercise: a review—Part III: Effects of nutritional interventions. *Int J Sports Med,* 1988 Aug;19(6):371–9.

4. Goforth, Jr, HW, et al. Persistence of supercompensated muscle glycogen in trained subjects after carbohydrate loading. *J Appl Physiol,* 1997 Jan;82(1):342–7.

5. McCarty MF. The origins of western obesity: A role for animal protein? *Med Hypotheses,* 2000 Mar;54(3):488–94.

CHAPTER 13

1. Kessler D. Cancer and herbs. *N Engl J Med,* 2000;342:1742–3.

2. Heinonen OJ. Carnitine and physical exercise. *Sports Med,* 1996 Aug;22(2): 109–32.

3. Villani RG. L-Carnitine supplementation combined with aerobic training does not promote weight loss in moderately obese women. *Int J Sport Nutr Exerc Metab,* 2000 Jun;10(2):199–207.

4. Cupp MJ. Herbal remedies: Adverse effects and drug interactions. *Am Fam Physician,* 1999 Mar 1;59(5):1239–45. Review.

5. Whybark MK. Dietary supplements: Are you getting what you pay for? *Today's Dietician,* 2002 Sept:42–44.

6. Bermejo Vicedo T, et al. Antioxidants: The therapy of the future? *Nutr Hosp,* 1997 May–Jun;12(3):108–20.

7. Mo JQ, et al. Decreases in protective enzymes correlates with increased oxidative damage in the aging mouse brain. *Mech Ageing Dev,* 1995 Jul 14;81(2–3):73–82.

8. Virtamo J, et al. Effect of vitamin E and beta carotene on the incidence of primary nonfatal myocardial infarction and fatal coronary heart disease. *Arch Intern Med,* 1998 Mar 23;158(6):668–75.

9. Dekkers JC. The role of antioxidant vitamins and enzymes in the prevention of exercise-induced muscle damage. *Sports Med*, 1996 Mar;21(3):213–38.

10. Sen CK. Antioxidants in exercise nutrition. *Sports Med*, 2001;31(13):891–908. Review.

11. Dekkers JC, et al. The role of antioxidant vitamins and enzymes in the prevention of exercise-induced muscle damage. *Sports Med*, 1996 Mar;21(3):213–38.

12. Chan AC. Partners in defense, vitamin E and vitamin C. *Can J Physiol Pharmacol*, 1993 Sep;71(9):725–31.

13. Stephens NG, et al. Randomised controlled trial of vitamin E in patients with coronary disease: Cambridge Heart Antioxidant Study (CHAOS). *Lancet*, 1996 Mar 23;347(9004):781–6.

14. Heinonen OP, et al. Prostate cancer and supplementation with alpha-tocopherol and beta-carotene: Incidence and mortality in a controlled trial. *J Natl Cancer Inst*, 1998 Mar 18;90(6):440–6.

15. Swain RA, et al. Therapeutic uses of vitamin E in prevention of atherosclerosis. *Altern Med Rev*, 1999 Dec;4(6):414–23.

16. Behrens WA, et al. Tissue discrimination between dietary RRR-alpha- and all-rac-alpha-tocopherols in rats. *J Nutr*, 1991 Apr;121(4):454–9.

17. Bendich A, et al. The health effects of vitamin C supplementation: A review. *J Am Coll Nutr*, 1995 Apr;14(2):124–36. Review.

18. Head KA. Ascorbic acid in the prevention and treatment of cancer. *Altern Med Rev*, 1998 Jun;3(3):174–86.

19. Ausman LM. Criteria and recommendations for vitamin C intake. *Nutr Rev*, 1999 Jul;57(7):222–4.

20. Packer L, et al. Neuroprotection by the metabolic antioxidant alpha-lipoic acid. *Free Radic Biol Med*, 1997;22(1–2):359–78. Review.

21. Lass A, et al. Electron transport-linked ubiquinone-dependent recycling of alpha-tocopherol inhibits autooxidation of mitochondrial membranes. *Arch Biochem Biophys*, 1998 Apr 15;352(2):229–36.

22. Casey A, et al. Metabolic response of type I and II muscle fibers during repeated bouts of maximal exercise in humans. *Am J Physiol*, 1996 Jul;271(1 Pt 1):E38–43.

23. Bemben MG, et al. Creatine supplementation during resistance training in college football athletes. *Med Sci Sports Exerc*, 2001 Oct;33(10):1667–73.

24. Häussinger D, et al. Cellular hydration state: An important determinant of protein catabolism in health and disease. *Lancet,* 1993 May 22;341(8856):1330–2.

25. Casey A, et al. Creatine ingestion favorably affects performance and muscle metabolism during maximal exercise in humans. *Am J Physiol,* 1996 Jul;271(1 Pt 1): E31–7.

26. Williams MH, et al. Creatine supplementation and exercise performance: An update. *J Am Coll Nutr,* 1998 Jun;17(3):216–34. Review.

27. Demant TW, et al. Effects of creatine supplementation on exercise performance. *Sports Med,* 1999 Jul;28(1):49–60. Review.

28. Poortmans JR, et al. Adverse effects of creatine supplementation: Fact or fiction? *Sports Med,* 2000 Sep;30(3):155–70. Review.

29. Schilling BK, et al. Creatine supplementation and health variables: A retrospective study. *Med Sci Sports Exerc,* 2001 Feb;33(2):183–8.

30. Hultman E, et al. Muscle creatine loading in men. *J Appl Physiol,* 1996 Jul;81(1):232–7.

31. Casey A, et al. Does dietary creatine supplementation play a role in skeletal muscle metabolism and performance? *Am J Clin Nutr,* 2000 Aug;72(2 Suppl): 607S–17S. Review.

32. Green AL, et al. Carbohydrate ingestion augments skeletal muscle creatine accumulation during creatine supplementation in humans. *Am J Physiol,* 1996 Nov;271(5 Pt 1):E821–6.

CHAPTER 14

1. Randall VA. Role of 5 alpha-reductase in health and disease. *Baillieres Clin Endocrinol Metab,* 1994 Apr;8(2):405–31.

2. Griggs RC, et al. Effect of testosterone on muscle mass and muscle protein synthesis. *J Appl Physiol,* 1989 Jan;66(1):498–503.

3. Wright JE. Anabolic steroids and athletics. *Exerc Sport Sci Rev,* 1980;8: 149–202.

4. Roth SM, et al. Muscle size responses to strength training in young and older men and women. *J Am Geriatr Soc,* 2001 Nov;49(11):1428–33.

5. Lee IM. Associations of light, moderate, and vigorous intensity physical activity with longevity. The Harvard Alumni Health Study. *Am J Epidemiol,* 2000 Feb 1;151(3):293–9.

6. Saitou N, et al. Evolution of primate ABO blood group genes and their homologous genes. *Mol Biol Evol,* 1997 Apr;14(4):399–411.

7. Martinko JM, et al. Primate ABO glycosyltransferases: Evidence for trans-species evolution. *Immunogenetics,* 1993;37(4):274–8.

8. Bodánszky H, et al. Incidence of lactose malabsorption in the population 6–18 years of age. *Orv Hetil,* 1990 May 13;131(19):1029–32.

9. Dohm GL, et al. Metabolic responses to exercise after fasting. *J Appl Physiol,* 1986 Oct;61(4):1363–8.

10. Coyle EF, et al. Fatty acid oxidation is directly regulated by carbohydrate metabolism during exercise. *Am J Physiol,* 1997 Aug;273(2 Pt 1):E268–75.

11. Davis JM. Weight control and calorie expenditure: Thermogenic effects of pre-prandial and post-prandial exercise. *Addict Behav,* 1989;14(3):347–51.

12. Goben KW, et al. Exercise intensity and the thermic effect of food. *Int J Sport Nutr,* 1992 Mar;2(1):87–95.

13. Nichols J, et al. Thermic effect of food at rest and following swim exercise in trained college men and women. *Ann Nutr Metab,* 1988;32(4):215–9.

14. Schabort EJ, et al. The effect of a preexercise meal on time to fatigue during prolonged cycling exercise. *Med Sci Sports Exerc,* 1999 Mar;31(3):464–71.

15. Williams MH. Facts and fallacies of purported ergogenic amino acid supplements. *Clin Sports Med,* 1999 Jul;18(3):633–49.

16. Silk DB, et al. Characterization and nutritional significance of peptide transport in man. *Ann Nutr Metab,* 1982;26(6):337–52.

17. Steinhardt HJ. Comparison of enteral resorption rates of free amino acids and oligopeptides. *Leber Magen Darm,* 1984 Mar;14(2):51–6.

18. Demont RG, et al. Comparison of two abdominal training devices with an abdominal crunch using strength and EMG measurements. *J Sports Med Phys Fitness,* 1999 Sep;39(3):253–8.

19. Frayn KN. Regulation of fatty acid delivery in vivo. *Adv Exp Med Biol,* 1998; 441:171–9.

20. Kraemer WJ. Detraining the bulked-up athlete: Prospects for a lifetime of health and fitness. *Natl Strength Cond Assoc J,* 1983;5:10–12.

21. Tucci JT, et al. Effect of reduced frequency of training and detraining on lumbar extension strength. *Spine,* 1992 Dec;17(12):1497–501.

22. Wolfe RR. Fat metabolism in exercise. *Adv Exp Med Biol,* 1998;441:147–56.

23. Tremblay A, et al. Impact of exercise intensity on body fatness and skeletal muscle metabolism. *Metabolism,* 1994 Jul;43(7):814–8.

24. Phelain JF, et al. Postexercise energy expenditure and substrate oxidation in young women resulting from exercise bouts of different intensity. *J Am Coll Nutr,* 1997 Apr;16(2):140–6.

25. Sedlock DA, et al. Effect of exercise intensity and duration on postexercise energy expenditure. *Med Sci Sports Exerc,* 1989 Dec;21(6):662–6.

26. Treuth MS, et al. Effects of exercise intensity on 24-h energy expenditure and substrate oxidation. *Med Sci Sports Exerc,* 1996 Sep;28(9):1138–43.

27. Lee VC, et al. Exercise and pregnancy: Choices, concerns and recommendations. In: *Obstetric and Gynecologic Physical Therapy,* New York, Churchill-Livingstone.

28. Clapp JF. The course of labor after endurance exercise during pregnancy. *Am J Obstet Gynecol,* 1990;163:1799–805.

29. Clapp JF. Morphometric and neurodevelopmental outcome at age five years of the offspring of women who continued to exercise regularly throughout pregnancy. *J Pediatr,* 1996;129(6):856–63.

30. Collis N, et al. Cellulite treatment: A myth or reality: A prospective randomized, controlled trial of two therapies, endermologie and aminophylline cream. *Plast Reconstr Surg,* 1999 Sep;104(4):1110–14; discussion 1115–17.

31. Rosenbaum M, et al. An exploratory investigation of the morphology and biochemistry of cellulite. *Plast Reconstr Surg,* 1998 Jun;101(7):1934–9.

32. Lotti T, et al. Proteoglycans in so-called cellulite. *Int J Dermatol,* 1990 May;29(4):272–4.

33. Draelos ZD, et al. Cellulite. Etiology and purported treatment. *Dermatol Surg,* 1997 Dec;23(12):1177–81.

34. Faust IM, et al. Adipose tissue regeneration following lipectomy. *Science,* 1977 Jul 22;197(4301):391–3.

35. Larson KA, et al. The effects of lipectomy on remaining adipose tissue depots in the Sprague Dawley rat. *Growth,* 1978 Dec;42(4):469–77.

36. Heaney RP, et al. Excess dietary protein may not adversely affect bone. *J Nutr,* 1998 Jun;128(6):1054–7. Review.

37. Holbrook TL. Calcium intake: Covariates and confounders. *Am J Clin Nutr*, 1991 Mar;53(3):741–4.

38. Patrick L. Comparative absorption of calcium sources and calcium citrate malate for the prevention of osteoporosis. *Altern Med Rev*, 1999 Apr;4(2):74–85. Review.

39. Eaton SB, et al. Calcium in evolutionary perspective. *Am J Clin Nutr*, 1991; 54:281S–7S.

40. Geinoz G, et al. Relationship between bone mineral density and dietary intakes in the elderly. *Osteoporos Int*, 1993 Sep;3(5):242–8.

41. Lacey JM, et al. Correlates of cortical bone mass among premenopausal and postmenopausal Japanese women. *J Bone Miner Res*, 1991 Jul;6(7):651–9.

42. Cooper C, et al. Dietary protein intake and bone mass in women. *Calcif Tissue Int*, 1996 May;58(5):320–5.

43. Munger RG, et al. Prospective study of dietary protein intake and risk of hip fracture in postmenopausal women. *Am J Clin Nutr*, 1999 Jan;69(1):147–52.

44. Barzel US, et al. Excess dietary protein can adversely affect bone. *J Nutr*, 1998 Jun;128(6):1051–3. Review.

Index

About the Author

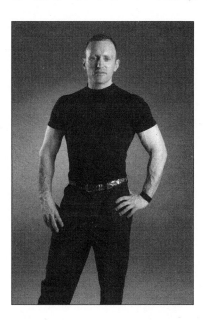

Brad Schoenfeld is widely regarded as one of America's leading health and fitness experts. He is the author of the top-selling fitness books *Look Great Naked*, *Look Great Sleeveless*, *Look Great at Any Age*, and *Sculpting Her Body Perfect*. He has been published or featured in virtually every major magazine (including *Cosmopolitan*, *Self*, *Marie Claire*, *Fitness*, and *Shape*) and has appeared on hundreds of television shows and radio programs across the United States. Certified as a strength and conditioning specialist (by the National Strength and Conditioning Association) and as a personal trainer (by both the American Council on Exercise and the Aerobics and Fitness Association of America), Schoenfeld was awarded the distinction of being classified as a Master Trainer by the International Association of Fitness Professionals. He is also the producer of three videos, which feature his Look Great program, and runs the Web site www.lookgreatnaked.com. A frequent lecturer on both the professional and consumer level, Schoenfeld is owner/operator of the exclusive Personal Training Center for Women in Scarsdale, New York. He lives in Croton-on-Hudson, New York.

NOW AVAILABLE ON VHS & DVD

Get the sleek, sexy silhouette you've always wanted... with the ultimate trouble-zone targeted videos.

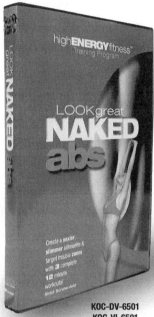

KOC-DV-6501
KOC-VI-6501

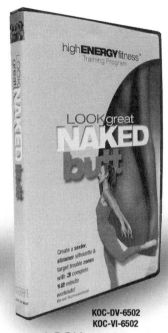

KOC-DV-6502
KOC-VI-6502

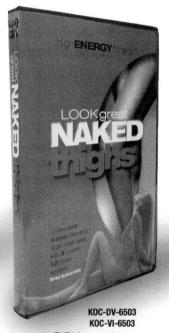

KOC-DV-6503
KOC-VI-6503

LOOK great
**NAKED
abs**

LOOK great
**NAKED
butt**

LOOK great
**NAKED
thighs**

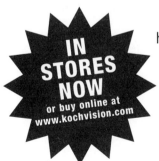

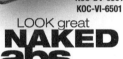

Experience the personal training expertise of *Brad Schoenfeld* right in your own home, with his best-selling video series *Look Great Naked*

Brad has specially designed these training programs to be time-efficient, with maximum results in a workout that fits into any schedule. Emphasis is placed on quality, not quantity, to bring you a highly effective targeted workout. Based on the best-selling book of the same title, Look Great Naked will tighten and sculpt your thighs, abs, and butt, and heighten your confidence. Even beginners will notice a difference in their muscle tone and energy level in just a few short weeks.

For health tips, contests & more fitness videos visit www.kochvision.com

KOCH VISION

© 2003 KOCH Entertainment, LLC. "Look Great Naked" is a trademark owned by Global Fitness Services and used under license.

Penguin Group (USA) Inc. is not associated with KOCH Entertainment, LLC, or Global Fitness Services, which are solely responsible for the information, services, and products offered herein.

Other Books by Brad Schoenfeld

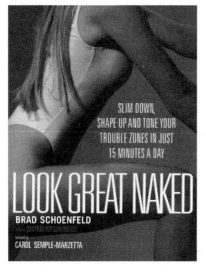

ISBN 0-7352-0230-3

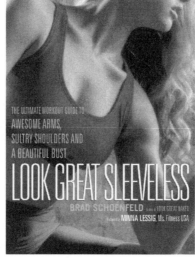

ISBN 0-7352-0304-0

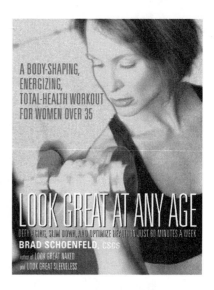

ISBN 0-73520-331-8